Eating to Win

"Useful to the athlete attempting to correct certain nutritional deficiencies, as well as to others wishing to increase strength and stamina." —*Library Journal*

"Emphasizes the always tantalizing topic of how to lose weight as well as how to improve your health as you shed those pounds." —*Playgirl*

"Informative ... down-to-earth knowledge for the concerned athlete .... Excellent." —*Whole Foods*

* * * * * * * * *

Frances Sheridan Goulart's articles on sports nutrition and cooking have appeared in *The New York Times*, *Redbook*, *Vogue*, *Runner's World* and many other publications. She's a long-distance runner; she swims; and she bicycles 4000 miles every year.

D0057305

EATING

TO

*W*IN

Food Psyching for the Athlete

Frances Sheridan Goulart

STEIN AND DAY / *Publishers* **/ New York**

FIRST STEIN AND DAY PAPERBACK EDITION 1984

FIRST STEIN AND DAY PAPERBACK EDITION 1984
Day Books edition 1982
First published in hardcover by Stein and Day/*Publishers*
   in 1978.

Copyright © 1978 by Frances Sheridan Goulart
All rights reserved, Stein and Day, Incorporated
Designed by Barbara Huntley
Printed in the United States of America
Stein and Day/*Publishers*
Scarborough House
Briarcliff Manor, N.Y. 10510
ISBN 0-8128-8095-1

*For MOM
and DAD,
who taught me
to eat
and run*

Note

This book deals with foods and related substances that provide energy, strength, and vitality to the human body. Any consideration of drugs that may do the same thing has been excluded since the author is not a medical person. If you think you'd like to follow any of the diets, take the vitamins or minerals, or pursue any other ideas presented in this book, you should consult your personal physician beforehand.

Contents

Eating to Win

1 / *Eating to Win*

"Anyone who enters athletics," says Dr. Otto Brucker, "announces indirectly that he is not interested in neglecting his body." This is true of even the casual athlete, and there are an estimated 87.5 million of those in America, not counting kids.

Of that number, eight million jog, twenty-nine million play tennis, fifty thousand are racquetball regulars, and almost half a million paddle on the paddle courts.

There are nearly fifteen million men and women over the age of 20 riding bikes these days and nearly forty-six million walking for health and recreation.

More than seven million adult Americans are downhill skiers, and uncounted numbers of us have also discovered the joys of skating, cross-country skiing, and the ball sports, including handball, volleyball, softball, and golf.

But a big part of not neglecting your body, besides exercise, has to do with food. You can eat to win if you know how, and this book will give you that know-how.

There are lots of ways to increase your energy, endurance, and stamina—things you need to improve your game.

You can experience a hormonal high without hormones, hard drugs, or hanky-panky. There are vitamin fixes, sweat fixes, carbohydrate fixes, honest "uppers" like megaminerals and natural side-effect-free stimulants like certain amino acids. And there is piggyback-nutrient-loading, combining vitamins that work synergistically in a matter of hours, days, or weeks to improve your health and vitality dramatically.

There is the safe "speed" that comes from ginseng, chia seeds, pollen, liver powder, and food yeast, both alone and in various combinations.

Odd as it may sound to those who haven't experimented with fasting, even *not* eating is another effective upper for many. "In common with salmon, people discover they have amazing resources of energy during and after fasting. When we lose a lot of weight, we are, naturally, going to feel more energetic because our strength isn't being sapped carrying around all that waste poundage." So says fasting authority Alan Cott.

Even turning the lights off, strange as it seems, can turn you on. The type of sleep necessary for super biological health and top performance occurs after exercise, studies show. By increasing protein synthesis, it provides you with speed, strength, and endurance.

Above all, foods—simple, inexpensive foods—spell the difference between just getting by and getting to the top of your form. If you've been down so long it looks like up to you, it's time for a change.

A switch, for instance, from quick-burning refined sugar to the natural sugar in natural foods like 99 percent calorie-and-cholesterol-free sprouts could be just what the coach ordered. Sprouts contain a high level of natural sugar because they are the most "alive" food known. They require little digestive breakdown and produce none of the nerve-shattering downs that sugars do.

Maybe you won't be able to leap tall buildings in a single bound after eating an organic banana, but you should be able to get off the ground and make your best a little better than before.

Nutritional mainlining made a new man out of Bobby Riggs; wonder foods and vitamins made a new champ out of Mohammad Ali, and with a combination of fasting, juicing, and raw foods, Dick Gregory recycled himself into the kind of lay athlete who could run marathons with the ease with which most folks walk to the mailbox.

Why not a new, more vigorous you?

Studies show that dietary control can improve endurance by 200 percent. Dietary adjustments can even influence your sweating rate, and by adding fresh fruit juices, fresh vegetables, and raw soups to your diet you can reduce your chances of exercise-induced heat stroke by as much as 50 percent.

A bare handful of bad habits account for the vast majority of the physical-performance losses caused by wrong fuels.

If we would get control of our lives as Gandhi has suggested, we must first get control of our palates. So, too, does any true revitalization of our sporting lives begin with the palate.

Whatever you decide to do, it's wise to proceed slowly. "If you change one bad eating habit every two months," advises cyclist George Beinhorn, who changed several himself, "you'll be doing spectacularly well."

The dean of the natural hygienists, Herbert Shelton, says it takes three to five years to change eating habits.

You cannot rush into dietary disciplines any more than

you can rush into a new sports program without warming up, without a breaking-in period.

And don't draw conclusions about the validity of any nutritional regime on the basis of a two-week trial. Says Paavo Airola in *Let's Live* magazine,

> First, any drastic change in nutritional patterns will usually result in an immediate change for the better—vegetarians changing to a meat diet experience improved well being, just as meat-eaters feel better when they change to a vegetarian diet. Second, not how you feel in two weeks, but in two years or fifty years is what matters. The long-range effect is the only truly scientific evidence that is acceptable when we deal with nutrition.[1]

But learning good nutritional habits is worth doing, because "Improving the quality of what you eat leads to more than just higher scores and faster racing," to quote *Food for Fitness.*[2] "Athletics brings new complexes of experience . . . similarly pure foods, fasting and regulating the amount you eat renew all your senses and deepen the quality of all your perceptions."

Now, having said grace, let's eat to win.

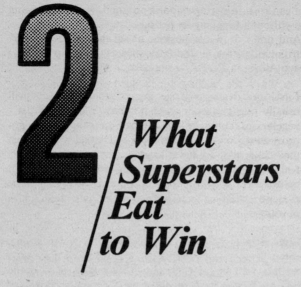

2 / What Superstars Eat to Win

Zero in on any minus food, one with negative consequences, and chances are you'll find a famous sports figure eating it, drinking it, or "loading it." There is considerable variance, to say the least, in the foods that sustain the "bionic" men and women among us and a woeful randomness with which many professional athletes augment their diets with vitamins and supplements.

The slapdash diet unfortunately is a commonplace in sports.

Jack Bacheler, a long-distance runner, is a good "bad" example. Jack goes in for carbohydrate loading and Coke. "During my marathon running, I will drink sixty-four ounces of uncarbonated Coke at intervals along the way. This seems to give me an additional kick."

In contrast, *Prevention* reports that Wayne Stetina,

champ racing cyclist, leisurely rolls out of bed and serves himself "a good dish of wheat germ and a liberal amount of vitamin E. . . . Fully awakened, he munches on some fruit, and finally mixes a bowl of millet, barley and rice for the main breakfast course. . . ."

Now that's the stuff of which the breakfast of champions *should* consist but rarely does.

A more typical eating pattern is that of crack long-distance runner Mary Decker. Her coach, Bob Glazier, observed, "I'll bet you can tell that's her room. Look at all that garbage. That kid's a regular garbage Disposall." Reporter Roberta Ostroof, picking up where Glazier left off, noted, "There are bags of mother's cookies, bags of bite-size Bit o'Honeys, chewing gum, Hostess Ding Dongs, and a coffeepot caked with spaghetti, sitting on a small plastic table top. . . ."

Are carbohydrate foods addictive? Ruth Adams's study of carbohydrates and obesity strongly suggests they are. She writes, [1] "There is convincing evidence that many modern foods high in carbohydrates tend to be far more fattening than even their high calorie content would indicate, because *they tend to make addicts out of people who consume them every day . . .*" [italics mine]. Mary Decker's meals seem to be an example of just such a junky starch and sugar diet that can be both habit-forming and health-damaging.

Then, there are the athletes who mainline mostly on nothing. Erik Ostbye, a senior marathoner from Sweden, thinks fasting for a few days before competing is the key to his good times (2:20 was one of them for the 26 mile-plus run). More on the less-than-less diet later.

Says Aldo Scandurra, another marathoner, "When I get up the day of the Boston Marathon, I don't eat at all. I take a large glass of hot water, have a bowel movement, and I'm ready for that race at noon"

And comedian-cum-runner Dick Gregory loves nothing more than a nice juicy run. In 1974, Gregory ran 900 miles in thirty days on nothing more than fruit juice.

Of course, everybody isn't spaced out on sugar donuts and Suzy-O's. Ballplayer Thurman Munson is partial to heavily-salted hard-boiled eggs. Tennis star Martina Navratilova likes strawberry shakes; Australian miler Herb Elliott breakfasts on walnuts, diced bananas, dried fruits, and raw oats.

In a recent survey of America's top cyclists, 68 percent indicated that they were "very conscious of their nutrition." As a group, cyclists tend to avoid junk foods, eat plenty of fresh fruits and vegetables, and take vitamin and mineral supplements. There are a lot of vegetarians in this sport, too.

Runner-rider-writer George Beinhorn, for example, eats "on yoga terms." "After a long run, there is no question about heading for the nearest store to get some fruit. I've found berries to be the most refreshing post-race food, especially strawberries and blueberries. Raw milk also seems to be a good recovery drink."

Norwegian runner John Systad, winner of eight championships, eats only fruit during most of the day and then consumes a dinner of "many onions, a raw and cooked potato, and two slices of whole grain bread."

For Billie Jean, it's protein and carbohydrates three times a day and no refined sugar or flour. Not that it comes easy. "She'd enjoy her meals a lot more with ten chocolate bars and a gallon of ice cream," confided fitness expert Joanne Taylor, who supervised a recent restyling of Ms. King's training and eating regimens

Jockey Mary Bacon admits to a sweet tooth, too, looking forward to what she calls a "high-pleasure dessert" after her customary low-calorie supper salad.

Golfer Carol Mann, however, would make an incompatible dinner partner for Jenner. By her own admission, she thrives on "laughter, gentle needling, and Brandy Alexanders."

British marathoner Ron Hill usually follows a high-protein and fat diet but switches over to a honey-heavy diet when competition is close at hand, eating honey not once or twice but four times a day. According to an observer, he wolfs down "great slices of whole-meal bread dripping with honey to furnish the glycogen needed by his exhausted muscles."

As for basketball great Ajrry Aclsu's three squares, they aren't. In the interest of fitness, he slashes it to one square, breakfast, and spends the other two meal times "running around a lot." Olympic gold medalist Frank Shorter runs around a lot but not till he's had a banana.

Jared Beads, an ultra marathoner (50 miles or more) who is given to road work of 25 miles a day during the week and twice that distance on weekends, says his training food consists of raw ground beef and raw eggs.

Even more interesting than the rations themselves may be the rationalizations given for what athletes eat.

Olga Korbut "chews gum to keep her rhythm going."

Ray Seales, a light-welterweight Olympic boxing champ, says, "I don't eat any bread or starch. It makes me soft inside."

Julius Erving avoids beans, milk, and too much soda "because they take their toll."

Bill Shoemaker is a big eater who'll eat what's put in front of him. He eats like a horse, of course!

Dorothy Hamill's training diet is almost faultless, consisting of granola and honey for breakfast, yogurt and fruit for lunch, meat and salad for dinner. She confesses, "I always have dessert, but so far they haven't inflicted any damage." And she makes her desserts herself; carrot cake and "wild ice cream things" are her favorites.

Arthur Ashe is sweet on sweet potato pie.

Similarly. Chris Evert's eating patterns are sensible and fit the medical profession's definition of a "mixed diet." There's breakfast always, followed by a small lunch and a big dinner. Breakfast usually consists of grapefruit, two eggs, one slice of whole-wheat toast, and maybe a slice of bacon. Her only borderline eccentricity is her attachment to honey, which she carries to the courts with her.

Dynamite runner Cheryl Toissant's only breakfast attachment is not to a croissant but to a cod-liver oil supplement and a multivitamin. Later, however, she brunches on oatmeal, juice, and toast or a high-protein meal of scrambled eggs, bacon, or steak and a vanilla malted. But it's never taken less than four hours before a track meet.

Many athlete's meals, of course, are part of an overall team diet. One such is Olga Korbut's. Coach Knysh and the team's medical adviser, Dr. Lydia Legonkova, describe the diet for the team as balanced but sparse. The gymnasts must have "plenty of protein." Eggs, milk, hearty soups, and Russian bread head the list of "Do's." Fresh fruit, which isn't always available to them, is highly favored, too.

To this conventional diet, Olga adds pistachio nuts and sometimes five apples a day for "energy boosters," and she washes everything down with sixteen glasses of milk daily. Olga also reportedly shares a passion with former President Nixon for tomato catsup.

What vitamin supplements do pro athletes take to augment their food supply?

Once again you might conclude you can be a winner on the courts, track, or field with vitamins or without. Bobby Riggs, for example, is a vitamin blitzer, reportedly taking as many as 415 a day before his court appearances. But superstar Mark Spitz turns in star performances without any vitamin supplements.

As for the stars' supplements:

Leonard Hilton, National Indoor Champion in the three-mile run: "I'm a strong believer in additional vitamins C, E, and B complex each day."

John Smith, world record holder for the 440-yard run, takes a multivitamin and a protein supplement every day. "I figure it's better to have too much than not enough," he reasons.

Deanne Wilson, American champion in the women's high-jump, takes twelve assorted vitamin and mineral pills every other day.

Dwight Stones, bronze medal winner in the high jump, takes multivitamins plus "additional C and E each day. I think these help me guard against colds and infections," he says.

Al Feurback. "Yes, I take most all the supplements including a time-released vitamin powder, wheat-germ oil, and protein pills."

Olympic swimmer Doug Northway takes multivitamins and "several salt tablets during my training program."

Weightlifter Russ Knipp: "I take a multivitamin and wheat-germ oil."

Less than half of the athletes questioned by writer Ellington Darden felt that a diet of well-balanced meals alone, without supplements, would provide them with the energy and stamina needed for strenuous competition.

So, the stuff that hits celebrities' training tables and the stuff that supplements it, is not always top-notch legal tender for the tummy.

But the good Lord gave some of us better bods than others. Some gifted individuals are more junk-proof than others, but why not use what *is* ingested as a guide to what *should* be ingested.

There is a long chain of factors that intervenes between

the guzzling of a Pepsi or a Perrier and a good or bad performance.

Age, some stress, good and bad genes, are all factors that you can't change, but food is one place where you *can* call the shots. Don't blow them as early as breakfast.

3 / Junk Food and What It Does to the Athletic Body

Just what is junk food?

It's coffee and beer. It's anything that serves no real nutritional purpose. It's anything that's been processed to death like white bread. Nearly anything with too much fat like bacon, anything with too much sugar like candy and soda, anything with too much salt like potato chips and pretzels.

How, specifically, do junk foods affect the civilian athlete like you? Are you affected more or less than your sedentary buddies?

First the good news:

For adults, the importance of avoiding refined foods varies from individual to individual. ... Individuals who are highly active physically can probably tolerate more refined food than others. Because of their activity they use up more calories, this means they eat more food, and have a better chance of getting enough of the lubricants they need (amino acids, vitamins and minerals, etc.)

So says the author of *Nutrition in a Nutshell.*[1]

Other nutritionalists are not quite so ready to let you off the hook.

"Some things," says Thomas Bassler, a marathon-running M.D, "seem evil: distilled alcohol, white sugar, white flour, hardened vegetable oils, etc. . . . Many examples of test animals killed with such foods can be found in the literature. . . . Even the egg, when powdered, can kill an animal after the animal is made deficient with a low vitamin diet." [2]

It's been estimated that 98 percent of the critical nutrients of many foods have been destroyed by one factor or another by the time it reaches your training table.

This "2-percent food" was 50 percent of our diet in 1970, a considerable increase from the 10 percent it made up in 1940.

To take a specific example, a typical TV dinner loses approximately 40 percent of its vitamin A, 100 percent of its vitamin C, 80 percent of its B, 55 percent of its vitamin E in the processing, says Frederic R. Senti of the U.S. Department of Agriculture (USDA).

Even fresh-from-the-market vegetables have only half the vitamin C and other vitamins they have when they're picked. In some foods the vitamins may be there but are unavailable to the body for other reasons. Cabbage, for instance, has most of its ascorbic acid tied up in the form of ascorbinogen. And even frozen vegetables lose half of their nutrients after six months in the deep freeze.

But it isn't just a question of low-vitamin diets and empty calories.

According to the Department of Agriculture, Americans spent over $16 billion on low-vitamin man-made foods in 1975, and this figure is expected to reach $23 billion by 1980.

A synthetic egg is a bad egg, a good example of how man-made foods shortchange and poison at the same time. These fakers contain ten times more sugar and starch than "the real thing," in addition to a number of very unhealthy and not very digestible chemicals. And fake eggs cost you almost twice as much.

A diet of such foods may even cost you your life. "Medical scientists report that many of the man-made foods lack the essential trace minerals found in natural foods and that the source of much synthetic food is petroleum. That petroleum causes cancer has been known to researchers for over 3 decades." [3]

At the very least, such foods don't contribute to your performing at your best.

In today's diet one must beware of chemical additives and also the residues of pesticides, and of the injections which are used in the breeding of certain animals such as chicken and beef. These substances can injure the cells, interfere with the enzymes necessary to normal cellular function and promote allergies, lead to storage of foreign substances in the liver, and interfere with the normal intestinal bacteria that are needed in digestion. [4]

Dr. William Philpot, a noted "new breed" psychiatrist in Oklahoma City, notes that "Junk foods create ... behavioral problems, too." (Are you having too many tantrums on the tennis courts?) "Symptoms like aggressive behavior, poor concentration, ... and hyperactivity are often traceable to food. . . ." The major villains, says Philpot, are candy bars, soft drinks, and pastries. Junk foods like these cause fluctuations in the blood-sugar level affecting the cortex, which is the part of the brain that, among other things, governs perception functions.

Jacqueline Verrett, author and Federal Drug Administration (FDA) scientist and also one of the FDA's harshest critics, says there is probably no function of the body which chemicals cannot affect:

In rats, a preservative, benzoic acid (used in a wide array of supermarket foods), was found to interfere with growth and in high doses to cause neurological disorders. MSG, which is one of the end products of the sugar-refining process, when fed to infant mice destroyed nerve cells in the hypothalmus of the brain. The sequestrant calcium disodium EDTA (widely used in quick-energy foods and drinks) has caused liver lesions in young rats and kidney damage in humans—Carageenan, a thickener chemically derived from seaweed, has produced ulcers in several species of animals. The flavoring ammoniated glycyrrhizin (licorice) has caused heart failure, hypertension, fatigue and edema in humans who consumed excessive amounts of food containing it. Brominated vegetable oils (BVO), used especially in carbonated beverages, has induced heart, liver, thyroid, testicle, and kidney damage or changes in test rats. Other chemicals have caused diarrhea, destroyed certain vitamins such as B_{12}, interfered with vitamin absorption, produced vascular changes, interacted with other substances in the body to cause damage and generally produced the gamut of biological reactions.[5]

Some foods are junkier than others. One way to determine at a glance how good or bad a food is, is to look at microbiologist Michael Jacobsen's simple but ingenious Nutritional Scoreboard. It rates hundreds of common everyday foods on a scale from 0 to 200. Foods are rated according to their supply of vitamins A, B₁, B₂, C, niacin, iron, calcium, protein, fiber, trace minerals and unsaturated fat, but not their artificial-ingredient content. "The public," Jacobsen explains "desperately needs a simple, easy guide to foods and nutrition." Using his system of plusses and minuses, you can rate virtually anything from canned tomato soup to fresh collard greens. Highest marks go to liver, broccoli, cantaloupe, kale, and turnip greens. And top-scoring beverages are orange juice and skim milk, followed by whole milk and tomato juice.

The lowest ratings go to the junkiest foods, which Jacobsen singles out as soft drinks, sugared coffee, milk chocolate, and brownies.

One of the more villainous examples of an "empty calorie" energy food is much commercial ice cream. "Ice cream lovers steadily ingest such goodies as ethyl acetate, (used as a dry cleaning fluid), piperonal (also as a louse killer), amyl acetate (also a solvent for oil paint), propylene glycol (used in germicides and paint removers), and other chemicals with every mouthful. Ice cream is also loaded with saturated fats and salicylates, highly allergenic substances that are ruled out of the diets of hyperactive children."

In addition, ice cream contains large amounts of refined sugar, and that includes even those that boast that "nothing artificial has been added."

It's a crying shame. You scream, I scream, why do we all still scream for ice cream? If you can't get through a whole hot summer of tennis without the stuff, why not make your own yogurt-based dessert (see recipe section).

If even that seems like too much trouble after a long hot day, here's a sixty-second substitute:

Peel and freeze ripe bananas. Break up two or three of

them and put them into the blender with milk, your favorite nutritional powders, an egg, vanilla extract, molasses or maple syrup or honey and buzz away. It makes a thick, cold shake if you can't wait for it to freeze up.

How about main-meal fast foods? Frankly, hot dogs and burgers and the buns they rest on aren't much better than most junk foods. Beginning with the bun, you'll find that it lacks many important nutrients since white flour is virtually milled to death. Each bun or slice of white bread is deprived of such essential minerals as iron and zinc, a large number of the trace minerals, and very essential "energy" vitamins such as B_6, pantothenic acid, and folic acid.

The final result, after milling, represents less than half of the wheat kernel's nutritive value. What's left is little more than starch and low-grade protein.

Such a slice of bread has only one-eighth of the protein found in 4 ounces of wheat germ. When it's called "enriched," that means that although some twenty-five known food elements are removed, only two or three are returned, and then usually only in synthetic form.

What's put back often compounds the trouble. There's frequently too much iodine, the wrong kind of iron, one that's hard to assimilate, and usually no copper (without copper, iron can't be utilized), plus suspect chemicals such as BHA, BHT, and EDTA.

In Russia, wheat bread still contains 16–18 percent of the grain's original protein. That's how it used to stack up here at the beginning of the century. According to author Barry Commoner, a slice of American white bread now needs to be supplemented with a slice of cheese to come up to its Russian counterpart in nutritional value.

As for the burger, the facts are equally disheartening. "After a meal of meat, the increase in heart rate regularly climbs to a 25–50 percent rise above the fasting level and persists in experimental subjects from 15–20 hours, to reach a total of many thousand extra heartbeats," says Dr. J. H. Kellogg. W. R. C. Larson, M.D., reports in the September 1977 issue of *Vegetarian Times* that "the heart of the habitual meat-eater beats 72 to 80 times a minute ... 15,000 extra heart strokes every 24 hours makes an appreciable strain upon the vital forces." Excess fat, especially from animal sources, says Ernst Van Aaken, can "lead to an overload of the liver and bilary system with an increase in blood fats, which in turn results in an impairment of the circulation, increased body weight ... and ultimately the promotion of arteriosclerosis. ...[6]

Natural hygienist Herbert Shelton provides a handy definition of a wholesome nonjunk food. "To be a true food," he says, "the substance eaten must not contain useless or harmful ingredients." That's a definition that certainly wipes out candy fashioned from propylene glycol, glacial acetic and methyl anthranilate, and corn chips preserved with butylated hydroxytoluene, a component of TNT. It should be enough to make you turn to natural peanuts and plain yogurt again.

Perhaps even worse is EDTA, a chemical chelator that may appear in a wide spectrum of manufactured foods without being announced on the label. According to a report in the June 1976 *American Journal of Clinical Nutrition,* EDTA prevents the body from using the iron it gets from other foods.[7] The authors of the study, examining the link between EDTA and iron deficiency, fed volunteers amounts of EDTA consistent with the amounts that might normally appear in a typical store-bought diet. Then they analyzed samples of blood from each volunteer to see how much iron it contained. Roughly half the iron in the food eaten was not absorbed because of the presence of EDTA. And the more EDTA added to the diet, the less the iron was absorbed. Since EDTA is present in unknown amounts in soda, beer, liquor, salad dressings, and a wide spectrum of commercial foods, your only protection, if you continue to "junk it up," is to take iron supplements, vitamin C (which makes iron more readily absorbable), and cross your fingers. Liquid junk foods may harm you, too. But we'll go into that later.

On the other hand, wholesome food can become unwholesome food without your even knowing it. Who would believe that a fresh Macintosh could be in the same junk-food league with many of the fast food burgers? Yet according to *Prevention* magazine,

An estimated 35 to 40 percent of all fresh apples are coated with a layer of wax. Fifty percent of fresh tomatoes are and about 75 percent of all cucumbers are also coated with the material. Now the Center for Science in the Public Interest is asking the FDA to insure that restrictions on the use of such waxes be strictly enforced ... [these] waxes have not been tested for carcinogenicity or other possible harmful effects.

"If additive interactions were studied intensively," claimed Robert Rodale, "faith in the safety of processed foods would erode even more rapidly than it has."

A final problem processed foods pose is that they are synthetically fortified. That's not only dangerous for the allergic athlete or the younger athlete who may be disposed to chemically caused hypertensive behavior, it cheats him, too. If it doesn't damage his health directly it certainly adds nothing to the diet that he relies on for his energy and sense of well-being.

For instance, instead of the more costly and more effective fish-oil-based vitamin A, a palmitic acid ester is used. The commercial substitute for B_2 is arrived at by treating riboflavin with chlorophosphoric acid. Both iron and manganese appear in their sulfate forms in refined foods, which involve the use of sulphuric acid, a chemical widely used in the preparation of paints, varnishes, ceramics, and as a fungicide.

In place of natural B_1, synthetic thiamin mononitrate is used, and instead of the B_6 complex, only one of the three-factor complex that chemists can mimic is used. And so it goes.

No athlete with even half-serious aspirations would accept a brass medal if he'd earned a solid gold one, so why should you accept chemical substitutions for vitamins in the cereals, snacks and breads that you eat?

As the National Academy of Science has warned,

Many chemical components of natural food products have been identified. It is likely however that even more have not. The great number of chemical substances discovered in any single food study itself reflects an almost endless variety of specific chemical compounds that remain to be discovered in the foods that make up the diet of man.

Of all the junk foods, of course, sugar takes the cake. Even if you're making a concerted effort to avoid sugar, you're bound to lose the battle in part. Not only has sugar consumption increased by one-third since the early 1900s, but as figures gathered by the Senate Select Committee on Nutrition and Human Needs show, control of our sugar intake has shifted from the hands of the consumer to the hands, or rather the machines, of the food processors.

Sugar is a main ingredient in foods as seemingly diverse as barbecue-style Shake'n Bake to nondairy creamers. Says Dr. Ira L. Shannon, director of the Oral Disease Research Lab at the Veterans Administration hospital in Houston:

We've lost discretionary control of our sugar intake. Most of the sugar we eat is coming from sources we're really not aware of. It's almost unbelievable where we're finding sugar in the grocery market.

... A look at product ingredients on supermarket shelves reveals the difficulty of finding almost any type of prepared food product without sugar in it. It's used not only in sweet baked goods, desserts, and soft drinks, but also in sauces, many baby foods, almost all fruit drinks, salad dressings, canned and dehydrated soups, pot pies, frozen TV dinners, bacon and other cured meats, some canned and frozen vegetables, most canned and frozen fruits, fruit yogurt, and breakfast cereals. If you eat a hot dog, there is likely to be sugar in the meat, in the ketchup or relish, and in the bun. [8]

"Just about every risk factor ever known to contribute to heart disease has been documented to be aggravated by the intake of sugar," say Dr. Robert Atkins. The doctor is on the side of super energy and is definitely opposed to sugar. "Americans are eating ten times as much sugar as they should," he believes.

Another good reason to exclude junk from a diet that is performance-specific is simply that sugar in all its forms, including raw or brown sugar, corn syrup, dextrose, glucose, and honey, tend to draw too much fluid into the gastrointestinal tract from other parts of the body. That causes a dehydration problem that may well affect your performance levels, say experts.

Few foods in fact are worse for the athlete and aspiring athlete. Sugar interferes with cell respiration and therefore with uptake of adequate oxygen, disrupts the hormonal level of the blood, and distorts the calcium-phosphorus relationship in the body.

A candy bar can throw the calcium-phosphorus level out of whack for as long as seventy-two hours. That's a long time for the calcium level, so crucial in the function of the heart muscle, to be disturbed.

Sugar is definitely linked to the production of kidney stones, allergies, diabetes, and heart disease. And it can be found in 80–90 percent of all refined foods.

There is evidence, according to nutritionist Dr. Jean Mayer, that the sugar-rich foods included in the carbohydrate-loading diets of so many distance runners, skiers, and cyclists may be the cause of their shortages of such necessary trace elements as chromium and zinc. Indeed, Dr. John Yudkin, the eminent British biochemist and author of an exhaustive study of the ills associated with sugar, *Sweet and Dangerous,* says that a high sugar intake may be the single most important factor in the production of artery-clogging blood fats. "If only a fraction of what is already known about the effects of sugar were to be revealed in relation to any other material used as a food additive," says Yudkin, "that material would be promptly banned."

Sugar lowers levels of two of the vital minerals most important to any athlete who works up a sweat: potassium and magnesium. These play an essential role in the functioning of the heart, brain, and all the muscles. The body needs these minerals to metabolize sugar properly. If they are not supplied by the foods eaten, and they usually are not, they will be taken from other parts of the body. That can lead to familiar malfunctions such as heartbeat irregularities, muscle cramps, and sweat-debt syndromes.

"Sugar replacements" may spell worse trouble. The safety of saccharin, a chemical sweetener five hundred times sweeter than sugar, in your prerace potion or loaders' brownie is in serious question. There's concern about what it does to the nervous system, the muscles, and the heart.

Saccharin is made from a sulfonizol, and, like drugs that contain the compound, it can start allergic and toxic reactions affecting skin, heart rhythms, and gastrointestinal tract, organs in which the athlete especially cannot afford dysfunctions. The American Association for the Advancement of Science found that saccharin caused more dangerous tumors in laboratory mice than do cyclamates; they believe it should be banned. As for glucose, several American nutritionists say that it is the only sugar absolutely known to provoke diabetes in test animals. Corn syrup is another unnatural sweetner. It's made by treating cornstarch with sulphuric acid, neutralizing it with sodium carbonate, and finally filtering it through beef bones to clarify it. Corn syrup has two aliases, commercial glucose and dextrose. It is cheaper than sugar and is assimilated even more rapidly than other sugars.

And what about the substitutes? Sorbitol, one of the postcyclamate alternatives, is a water-soluble powder derived from berries and other fruits. At the present writing, the FDA has not decided whether it is really safe for the diabetics for whom it is supposedly intended in soft drinks, candies, chewing gum, and other products. It has already been shown to cause digestive upsets and diarrhea at certain dose levels. And there is a suggestion that it may alter the way other medications that a person is taking are absorbed, too.

Then there is the newest of the sugar analogs, xylitol. Made from fruits and vegetables, it's claimed by its Norwegian producers to have a sweetness similar to that of sugar. It is twice as sweet as sorbitol, although its flavor is not sugarlike. The good news is that it may even fight tooth decay, but the bad news is that at certain dose levels, like all chemicals, it causes gastrointestinal distress and may even turn out to be a weak carcinogen like saccharin, something current British studies are suggesting.

Fructose or fruit sugar is also new; its value is vigorously attacked and defended by eminent authorities. Unlike the two preceeding substitutes, it can be bought now in tablets or in powdered form at approximately three dollars a pound. Looking very much like white refined sugar, it is less sweet and has good dissolving properties. It is to be sprinkled on your cereal or spooned into your coffee or tea. According to Carlton Fredericks, a report published in Britain's medical magazine *Lancet* said the scientific literature does not confirm its safety. Fructose is metabolized in the liver, where it causes increased lactate production, high-energy phosphate depletion, increased uric acid formation, and inhibition of protein synthesis. This raises blood lactate and serum uric acid to undesirable levels. In disorders involving the liver or lack of oxygen in the tissues, infusion of fructose can lead to a serious metabolic disturbance, lactic acidosis.

On the other hand, Dr. Robert Atkins, one of the chief defenders of fructose as an energy source and sugar substitute, says,

> Fructose is a simple sugar. To be metabolized, fructose, unlike glucose, does not require or call forth insulin. Thus it provides a readily available carbohydrate source for energy but one which does not evoke the insulin overresponse that characterizes the person with low blood sugar and is the most common cause of fatigue.

But there are other objections. Dr. Theron Randolph, perhaps the country's leading specialist on food and environmental allergies, says the name "fructose" is misleading. "Fructose, formerly referred to as 'fruit sugar,' is now made from cornstarch ... [and] allergy to corn is the leading cause of allergy in this country...."

So if you try it and find that rather than relieving your fatigue, fructose increases it, you may be one of the legion of those who are corn sensitive.

Nor does Dr. John Yudkin feel that fructose belongs in your daily tea or on your morning toast. "Many of the harmful effects of sucrose are due to the fructose component," he says. (The average 140-gram intake of sucrose yields about 70 grams of fructose.)

And according to a report in the *Journal of the American Medical Association,* "Fructose in excessive quantities may be converted to excessive amounts of sorbitol which the Russians consider to be a possible factor in the eye hemorrhages which are frequent in severe diabetes. . . ." The same magazine says that "fruit sugar in large amounts can worsen low blood sugar quite as efficiently as sucrose can."

Meanwhile, writing in Great Britain's *Athletic Weekly,* M. H. Arnold enthusiastically endorses fructose in its liquid form. "Fructose is rapidly and completely converted into glycogen. The speed of conversion is startling . . . to build up glycogen stocks, eat fructose. . . . Fructose has the unusual property of increasing the speed at which glucose is converted into glycogen—thus giving a kind of bonus."

Dr. Atkins, the advocate of fructose, offers these suggestions for using it in your diet:

Fructose can be taken in several ways. You can take two fructose tablets (2 grams each) every two hours. . . .

Or you can make lemonade with it, using about six teaspoons to a quart, and drink it throughout the day.

Or you can use fructose as you would ordinary sugar. To get the full antihypoglycemia effect, you may need a teaspoon or two of fructose each hour, which effectively curtails insulin release. Or you may need to use it only certain times of the day. Test it for yourself, watching for that point at which you might feel an energy letdown. If you feel fatigue, tension, or uneasiness, then you know it's time to take fructose again. . . .

You can use fructose in any recipe calling for sugar.

Just remember that fructose is two-thirds again sweeter than sugar. So if 5 teaspoons of sugar are called for, you need only 3 teaspoons of fructose.

Caution: Watch your triglycerides. Many investigations, despite Dr. Palm's studies, have found that fructose can raise the level of triglyceride in the blood. If you stay on fructose, make sure to test your triglyceride level. . . .[9]

For best effects fructose should be taken with the mineral magnesium, for maximal uptake.

Do not make the mistake of assuming that fructose is the same as the sugar in fruit or juice. Fruit sugar is actually half glucose and has the effect of stimulating rather than pacifying your insulin response.

Is it true or false that fructose is the sugar substitute we runners, rowers, swimmers, and weekend tennis players have been waiting for to replace our pocket Life Savers and between-meal Marathon Bars? You'll have to be an experiment of one until further damning or redeeming evidence comes in.

In the meantime, the question persists, Is there any way around the sugar cube? Yes, you can cycle, kick, stroke, row, or run your way right around the sugar cube and get squarely the other side of it. You can have an upper alimentary canal, esophagus, and duodenum that is non-ulcerated and unirritated by the sugar that, even in small doses, increases stomach acidity by 20 percent.

This sort of sugar-induced dither is no good for your inner game of tennis, soccer, or anything else. So what is the alternative?

Use less sugar or none at all. Use "natural" sweeteners like the following instead:

Honey

Feel like you're coming unglued? Reach for the honey, like Chris Evert does. Honey is an important antifatigue food since it is predigested, builds up the alkaline reserves in the blood and tissues and provides a maximum of energy with a minimum of shock to the digestive system. Sugar-laden foods overload the bloodstream in fifteen minutes; honey is absorbed over a period of four hours.

Honey is one of the oldest foods known to man. Authors Beck and Hedley unabashedly call it nature's number-one food in their book *Honey and Your Health*.[10]

To P. E. Norris, it is "nature's genuine energizer." Says he, "There is no energy-producing food on the market to touch honey. Nor will there ever be. All synthetic glucose products are inferior to honey not only for the speed with which honey brings about a sense of well-being but also for the production of real lasting energy and the alkalinizing of the body."

Honey contains more genuine fructose (39 percent) than any other comparable sweetener. (Real fructose or fruit sugar is also known as levulose.)

In addition to protein from the pollen, the substance responsible for the clouding in unfiltered honey, good honey contains some vitamin A, several vitamins from the B complex, and vital enzymes and minerals, such as phosphorus, potassium, calcium, sodium, sulphur, iron, magnesium, and manganese, all in the right small amounts and balance to serve the needs of the normal individual. Honey has antiseptic and hygroscopic properties, which means it draws moisture from anything it comes in contact with, including harmful microorganisms. No disease germs can survive in honey over a few hours.

It is a magical sort of foodstuff. It cannot be imitated or manufactured by man. There is something in its qualities that eludes science. And honey skeptics often forget that all honeys are not the same.

First of all, refined honey, or any honey not labeled "raw" and "unfiltered," is worthless since it has been cooked, strained, and often has white sugar and water added to arrest crystallization. Second, raw honeys differ from one another just as the flowers that lead to them do. Their smell, nourishing value, and healing powers depend (says honey expert P. E. Norris) on rain, sun, mineral content of the soil, on whether the plant is grown in humus or artificial fertilizer, and so on.

Honey eaters of some athletic fame include Sir Edmund Hilary, who scaled Mount Everest. Hilary, in private life, was a New Zealand bee farmer.

The sweet is a staple of the Indian wrestling-training diet: Such delicacies as labri, ludoos, and saundaesh are all made with honey, in combination with other high-powered fitness foods, that is, yogurt, raw cream, and unrefined molasses.

Honey is another of the nontoxic "uppers." "We do not use any stimulant except weak tea with a tablespoon of honey per cup. After a 20- or 30-mile hike a pint of this pick-me-up revives us completely in 15 to 20 minutes," say the mountain-climbing authors of *The Lords of the Rockies,* Wendell and Lucy Chapman.

And it is indisputable that athletes have found it "quicker than likker" since the beginning of time. Ancient Greek athletes used it as a training food, and Barbara Cartland, in *The Magic of Honey,* [11] describes the arrival of Russian athletes at the 1948 Olympic Games loaded down with steaks and honey. In 1936, the U.S. Public Health Service listed the energy value of a "gill" of honey as the equivalent of thirty eggs.

If you are pushing forty, fifty, sixty, note that honey seems to be the perfect instant food to prevent aging. A recent Russian study found that of two hundred people who were authenticated as being between 110 and 150, nearly all were or had been beekeepers and were all enthusiastic honey eaters.

According to Dr. Arnold Lorand, author of *Old Age Deferred,* "As the best food for the heart I recommend honey. ... It is easily assimilated and digested; it is the best sweet food. ... Before and after muscular exertion it should be given in generous doses. ..."

When you buy, buy it raw, and remember, the darker it is, the more nutrients you are getting for your money. Ideal storage temperature is about 72 degrees.

Unsulphured Molasses

This is not a by-product of the sugar-making process but a deliberately manufactured food, made from the juice of sun-ripened cane. It is also known as first-extraction molasses.

Unsulphured molasses imparts a taffylike flavor to baked goods, but if more than a quarter cup of sweetness is called for in a recipe, molasses may be a poor choice. Baked goods made with molasses stay moist and keep longer than sugar-sweetened foods.

Bypass sulphured molasses because it is a by-product of sugar making, a process in which noxious sulphur fumes are used; hence, the name.

Nutritionally, a better molasses is "blackstrap," which is the result of 30 gallons of cane juice boiled down to produce a single gallon of concentrated nectar. The sugar is then crystallized out and removed. For every ton of sugar made, there remains 30 gallons of blackstrap molasses, which contain all the minerals and heat-stable vitamins in the original cane.

This sweetener contains thirty times more nutrients than cane sugar. It has 58 mg. calcium in five tablespoons, more iron than eggs, and more potassium than any other food. It is an effective remedy for anemia and constipation because of its high levels of inositol, a B vitamin, and for some forms of arthritis because of the "Wurzen factor," which is also part of its nutritional makeup.

Maple Syrup

"Pure" maple syrup is an outstanding source of potassium and calcium and is also rich in sodium and phosphorus. About 40 gallons of maple sap are required to make 1 gallon of syrup, which explains its high price. Although Vermont and maple syrup are synonymous in the public mind, New York State, Ohio, and Quebec also rank high as producing regions. Nutritionally, syrup from Canadian sources is your best bet since bacterial and antifoaming agents are often used during processing in this country in addition to formaldehyde pellets to keep tap holes open. Most Canadian brands are processed without pellets.

In addition there are also these natural sweeteners: carob powder and carob syrup, sorghum syrup, date syrup and date sugar, and barley malt extract.

Note, too, that many foods (bread, cashew nuts, peanuts, potatoes, squash, and other nuts grains and vegetables will sweeten themselves if toasted. (This is dextrinization.) If you reduce fruit juice by boiling to a quarter or even less of its total volume, the natural sweetness will be concentrated, and you can even produce or heighten sweetness simply by freezing a food. (A banana from the freezer tastes like custard ice cream.)

Why not make your own sugar? Using raisins, for instance.

Just cover 1½ pounds of unsulphured raisins with twice as much water (currents may also be used), simmer twenty minutes, squeeze well, and strain. Makes 3 cups of raisin fructose.

Salt

A discussion about a junk food like sugar usually leads to questions about salt. Is salt something you can number among the "clean energy foods"?

It's true that athletes or near-athletes will occasionally need to add extra salt to their diets. Salt is necessary when you are near collapse from heat prostration, at which critical point plain water will, in fact, be useless. What you need when you are down and out is a 3 percent salt solution, since water will further dilute your rapidly escaping electrolytes (minerals). But fatigue short of this critical state is probably worsened by salt despite the folk tales.

Some experts say that replacement of sodium, when necessary, is probably best accomplished by means of timed-release sodium tablets, such as were used to advantage by the British football team in periods of great heat during the 1968 Olympic Games in Mexico.

But according to Dr. John Mann of the Bureau of Preventable Disease Control, N.Y. Department of Health, salt tablets are not advisable even in extreme heat. You can "O.D." on them, Mann states flatly.

The main electrolytes lost during physical exertion in hot weather, according to the Aerobics Institute (and their conclusions match those arrived at by the other respected studies), are not sodium but potassium and magnesium.

Remember, too, that salt intake contributes to low blood sugar and lower energy reserves by causing a further dip in blood potassium levels. This sets the stage for stress and for the retention of more salt and water.

In addition to those drawbacks, ordinary table salt is just as much a junk food as the junk foods it's sprinkled on.

According to Dr. Alan Nittler, "Regular table salt has been treated to extremely high temperatures which cause a physical change in the sodium nucleus structure so that it is no longer a substance that the body can use."

George Crane, author of "The Ocean's 44 Trace Minerals," says table salt is almost totally lacking in the many trace minerals found in natural unrefined salt. According to Crane, zinc, potassium, magnesium, and forty-one other trace minerals are refined out, leaving a product that is almost 100 percent sodium chloride, the stuff that raises so much cardiovascular Cain.

This is how it happens: Sea salt is produced by evaporating sea water in large ponds. The sun begins to concentrate the brine, and the first salt to crystallize out is sodium chloride. This is what is scraped off the top by refiners, then washed and dried by a nutrient-damaging heat process, leaving all the good stuff behind, as in most food processing.

This refined salt, according to other concerned researchers like Frank Wertz, now lacks potassium, which when in proper balance with sodium in the body helps to regulate the heartbeat. But a diet high in refined salt presents a serious risk of muscle damage and high blood pressure.

Salt has additives, too. It is usually "enriched" with iodine (synthetic) plus dextrose (sugar) to stabilize it, sodium bicarbonate to keep it white, and a chemical anticaking agent to keep it free flowing. (Kosher salt is just as treated, just as refined.)

What makes "whole salt" or "sea" salt of value is that it has almost the same balance of sodium chloride to minerals as that found in sea water. "This corresponds to the ratio of sodium chloride and minerals in human blood," says Wertz.

So sodium can be a real superstresser, not the tasty therapeutic wonder you may have heard. The sodium component of table salt also sucks excessive water from the tissues, forces the heart and kidneys to work harder than necessary, increases damage to the cirrhotic or chronically diseased liver, and in the opinion of some experts, brings on hypertension and can be particularly dangerous for an athlete over fifty-five.

According to studies by the National Research Council of the National Academy of Sciences, salt levels of as little as 2.8 percent of the diet of rats were "frankly hypertensigenic and life shortening." Although we are rat racers, not rats, it is significant that the salt in our human diet makes up an almost corresponding 2 percent.

According to Canadian P. Prioreschi, it is mineral imbalance that is the real culprit in causing heart disease, and his worldwide studies point to salt as the cause of this metabolic derangement. Salt, to his way of thinking, is a dangerous cardiotoxic agent, like alcohol and tobacco.

But on the opposite side of the salt question, low sodium reserves can spell fatigue, drowsiness, and depression. "The normal kidney excretes sodium without difficulty," claims Dr. H. L. Newbold, "and defects in the sodium metabolism (that is to say, some people are 'salt dumpers') may be as common as faulty carbohydrate metabolism."

"Salt is necessary. We have to have the chloride because it is part of hydrochloric acid. People who are low on adrenal functions also have a need for salt," agrees W. D. Currier.

Salt stimulates the production of hydrochloric acid in the stomach and in that respect is of some value to the aging athlete. But for most people, since the body under ordinary conditions needs no more than 1 gram per day and probably gets twice that amount just from natural foods, salt is a habit worth shaking. (Estimates are that the average American takes in between 10 and 15 grams of salt a day.)

According to the USDA's *Composition of Foods* book, 100 grams of potato chips, for instance (that's only 3 ounces), yield as much as 1000 mg. of sodium!

At levels like these, there is imminent danger of what Dr. Henry Beiler calls "salt poisoning." Hygienist Herbert Shelton, too, says salt is not a pepper-upper but a poison. "How can salt be a food when it passes through the body unchanged?" he asks. Marathoners have gone the distance trained without a trace of sodium chloride in their diets, and Shelton reminds us that both the American Indians and Rommel's North African troops got by nicely without salt.

In summary, having zeroed in on some of the mighty minus foods, the question remains, How can a junk food habit be broken or at least rerouted?

One method that works is fasting. According to Alan Cott, "When anyone abstains from food, profound changes take place. These changes revise attitudes about food and put appetite into alignment with the body's real needs for energy." One of the reasons people have for fasting as listed by Cott, is "to rid themselves of a junk-food past."

You can put your junk-food past behind you, too, if you try.

Read on.

4 / Superfoods for Super Performances

The circumstance of sports, even at the lay or weekend level, calls for a special combination of foods. What, then, about the reputation of those foods reputedly so essential for the health and energy of the athlete? In general, the "foods of fitness" will get some long-overdue scrutiny here, as well as the "wonder foods"—ginseng, pollen, etc.

In certain cases, a food will be classified as a "food for fitness" in one state and a "superfood" in another. Seeds are the perfect example of a fine fitness food in their un-germinated bean, nut, or grain state, which become "wonder foods" once they are sprouted.

Similarly, milk, regarded by some as a nearly perfect protein food (second only to the egg), becomes more perfect when cultured into yogurt. Now it is both a good food and a medicine that improves cholesterol levels and digestion, normalizes weight, increases longevity, and provides even more protein and B vitamins than it did in its fresh liquid state.

So let us begin with dairy products. Of the thirty-five most consumed foods in the United States, milk and cream are tops. Average per capita consumption was 291.2 pounds in 1975.

Yet how can anything that incites arthritis, sets the stage for atheriosclerosis, harbors salmonellosis, and provokes calcium deficiency, ironically enough be called a fitness food?

Such are the facts, however, about pasteurized, homogenized, modern milk.

And similar contradictory situations exist for other foods you have undoubtedly been brought up to regard as "foods for fitness," foods without which you would barely be able to get to first base, let alone steal second.

On the other hand, foods with bad reputations often have good points. Coffee, for instance, is a source of two prime sports-specific nutrients, the B vitamin niacin and the mineral magnesium. However, coffee's long list of negatives outweigh those positives.

"When you feed pasteurized milk to animals," says W. D. Currier, "they deteriorate." [1] And according to endocrinologist and author Henry Bieler,

> Milk is one of the most unstable thermolabile of all the natural foods. Even refrigeration for 24 hours will rob it of some of its vitamin content and its organic structure. Pasteurization disintegrates it even more, while boiling reduces it to a useless putrefiable mess that is tolerated by the liver with great difficulty ... certified raw milk when available should always be used.[2]

Nutritionist C. E. Burtis adds that lysine, one of the most important of the amino acids in protein foods, is damaged by heat, and this results in the body being unable to utilize other amino acids. The end product is incomplete metabolism.

A number of things appear to be wrong with pasteurization. One, a key enzyme, phosphate, needed to split and assimilate mineral salts in foods in the form of phytates, is destroyed. Two, protein is denatured, and its digestibility is reduced by 4 percent, its biological value by 17 percent. A great deal of calcium is lost, as well as 38 percent of the B vitamin complex, plus varying amount of C and A.

Even in its "raw certified" state there are some unnatural things about this "natural" food. As Dr. Ralph Bircher points out, the amino acid balance of cow's milk is a far cry from that required for optimal nutrition. Goat's milk, if you can't kick the bottle, is much closer to the ideal.

Dr. Nanna Swartz, professor of internal medicine at Stockholm's Karolina Institute, even warns that the bacteria found in milk and cheese may cause rheumatoid arthritis as well as other diseases. A bacteria called *Streptococcus B* remained after milk was pasteurized, she found, because it was more resistant to heat than the more common varieties of strep.[3]

Milk seems even less good as a pre- or postgame juicer when you get down to the grass roots. "Cows fed with fodder that has been subjected to insecticides and herbicides," says *Organic Gardening Magazine,* "may produce milk contaminated with residues of these chemicals that pasteurization does not eliminate."

Milk has its defenders, however. According to the author of *Milk and Milk Products in Human Nutrition,* "Only the whole carcass of an animal, including the bones and the liver, could contribute as much as milk, taken as a single food. Some people, such as the nomadic M'Bororo of West Africa, live for months exclusively on milk." Milk and butter also promote synthesis of vitamin B_6 in the intestines, thus contributing to a healthy heart and preventing cholesterol deposits, according to other experts.

And Adelle Davis, one of its staunchest proponents, emphasized that the vitamins in milk are in admirable harmony, at least the major ones, such as A, B $_2$ and C and D.

And milk-free diets are likely to be seriously deficient in riboflavin. (Milk supplies 45 percent of the riboflavin in this country's diet.)

So maybe you shouldn't be too quick to put milk out to pasture, after all, if it agrees with you—which brings up another problem. Dr. H. L. Newbold says:

> The inability to metabolize milk and dairy products runs as high as 40 percent even among adult Caucasions. Most children at about age 2 experience a gradual reduction of the body supply of lactase which is essential for digesting milk sugar. Studies at John Hopkins University revealed that up to 70 percent of Afro-Americans cannot metabolize milk properly.

Milk intolerance is a very common and often unsuspected cause behind the nausea, diarrhea, headaches, and sinus and cerebral dysfunctioning experienced by many of us jocks. But there's a good reason why you might find it hard to believe that milk like meat is not a fitness food.

These two industries together make up a $50 billion a year operation in the United State, and the dairy industry alone, with its 500,000 members, has many prominent people pushing milk.

If you are milk intolerant and still reluctant to give it up, there is another solution. You may find the answer is spiking your milk with a *milk digestant*, sold at health-food stores. Taken before a milk snack, this powder or tablet supplies the enzyme lactase, plus rennin, a natural digestant; it may allow you to enjoy your moo juice in peace.

But there are other problems even if you surmount the problems of pasteurization and lactase intolerance.

According to Dr. Kurt Oster of Park City Hospital in Bridgeport, Ct. something called xanthine oxidase in milk can cause certain phospholipids of the heart and arterial walls to oxidise into fatty acids that may later form atherosclerotic placques. Unfortunately, the homogenizing of milk makes xanthine oxidase all the more readily absorbed from the milk's fat globules. And unfortunately further, the sale of the vitamin folic acid, which helps to inhibit this unhealthy process, is severely restricted by our government's FDA. Dr. Oster recommends, as an at-home safety measure, heating milk to a boil to denature this enzyme.[4]

Fortunately, there are a number of alternatives to milk. Yogurt and other fermented milk products are free of most of the objections to milk. And then there are nuts. The average milk maven may not even suspect that there is as much calcium in a cup of Brazil nuts as there is in a glass of milk, and a cup of almonds supplies even more of this mineral. Even three dried figs are 35 percent calcium.

Sesame seeds are 60 percent oil, 18 percent protein, and one of the best sources of calcium this side of a cow's udder (1,125 mg. per 100 grams). And they can be used to make a highly palatable noncholesterol milk substitute.

You do not have to give up your wicked, wicked milky ways altogether; if you like the taste of milk, there remains something even better, one of the finest foods of fitness: yogurt and the whole family of fermented milks, which include kefir, acidophilus, buttermilk, even just plain clabbered or soured milk and of course the afore-mentioned yogurt.

Of course, the yogurt or fermented milk product you make yourself will be a far cry nutritionally from the kind you buy in the supermarket.

Most commercial yogurt has synthetic lactic acid added even when it isn't loaded up with sugary preserves which probably negate any good that might have come of the yogurt in its unsweetened state. Yogurt, you know, is *supposed* to be slightly tart.

But whichever kind you use, eat it up in a week's time, for the greatest good.

Yogurt is the stomach's soul food. It is the ideal medium for the absorption of protein. It doubles the intestinal absorption of calcium. The "friendly bacteria" in yogurt hinder the development of almost every disease-producing organism known, including those that change nitrites into nitrates plus salmonella and dysentery. (If you're going to keep eating those nitrate-filled ballpark hot dogs maybe you ought to at least have a cup of homemade yogurt to wash them down.)

Yogurt also increases the biological value of milk's protein and stimulates liver and intestinal activities.

Furthermore, yogurt is more rapidly digested than milk, over 90 percent of it in an hour. Whole milk takes two-thirds longer. Yogurt also manufactures a multitude of B vitamins (the energy complex again) in your digestive tract. As Karen Cross Whyte relates in *The Complete Yogurt Book,* "Ilya Metchnikoff identified and isolated the bacilli that did create yogurt, thus making it possible to process the food on a large scale. He gave the food the label 'health food,' stating that if a man ate yogurt regularly he would live to be one hundred fifty years old."

Animals fed yogurt every day live more than 10 percent longer than those on a yogurt-free diet, said Dr. Tomotari Mitsuoka of the Institute of Physical and Chemical Research in Japan, theorizing further that man would live 50 percent longer if his intestines were kept as close to sterile as possible. This is impossible, but eating lots of intestine-cleansing yogurt every day is both pleasant and possible for us all.

Even if winning the Boston Marathon at the age of ninety isn't what you're shooting for, still keeping your gut in good repair is simplified considerably by the addition of some sort of yogurt to your diet.

And Adelle Davis swore that in times of sickness, a quart of yogurt a day will put you back on your feet.

Advanced yogurt eaters may want to move up to such fermented milks or milklike products as kefir (a sort of super buttermilk), acidophilus, and "piima," a Finnish yogurt culture that requires no preboiling of the milk. All of these are carried by well-stocked health food shops.

Eggs

If milk has been overpraised as a food for fitness, eggs, whose per capita use declines each year, have probably been undervalued. Researcher Richard Passwater, for one, wonders what the nonegg eater is going to do for trace minerals like sulphur and selenium, for B vitamins, iron and lecithin, and for those other "phantom factors" in natural foods that spell the difference between passable health and peak states of well-being. And athletes who don't eat eggs at all, according to Dr. Carl C. Pfeiffer, of Princeton's Brain-Bio Center may be suffering from a serious lack of the trace mineral sulphur. Pfeiffer believes that this may be one reason for the widespread occurrence of arthritis—simply that arthritics do not eat enough eggs to get the right amount of sulphur they need for the health of the joints.

The Rodale *Natural Breakfast Book* calls eggs the most nearly perfect protein food: "Eat several eggs a day and you are treating yourself to nutritional excellence that is difficult to duplicate."

The white of an egg is 10 percent protein, the yolk is 16

percent, and between them they have a better distribution of amino acids, the basic components of protein, than any other food. Eggs offer the most concentrated amounts of protein for building and maintaining body tissue. Eggs lack vitamin C but not much else. They are low in calories, but their fat and protein content give the eater a feeling of satisfaction not always found in other low-calorie fare.

As a natural source of vitamin D, they are second only to cod liver oil.

And then of course, there is that tempest in an eggshell, the cholesterol controversy.

"Egg yolks," says the *Encyclopedia for Healthful Living,* "are known to be very high in cholesterol, but they are also high in lecithin and B vitamins both of which are used by the body in properly disposing of cholesterol. . . ." It further states that "the cholesterol that the body manufactures does not collect in the arteries nor does the cholesterol which comes to us from natural foods. It is the cholesterol we receive from processed foods which is the cause of our trouble."

Anyway, says Dr. Hans Fisher of Rutgers University, "People don't have to avoid foods containing fat and cholesterol if other foods they eat give their bodies a chance to cope with the problem and if they also exercise to a reasonable extent." [5]

Gerontologist Richard Passwater, whose research on cholesterol and the heart led to a book on the subject, says, "It has now been established that eating cholesterol does not cause heart disease, that muted cells within the artery walls form the atherosclerotic plaque and that certain nutrients can prevent both plaque formation and the fatal blood clots caused by plaques."

It is interesting, Passwater notes, that when *Science,* the official magazine of the American Association for the Advancement of Science, reviewed heart-disease research in its November 1976 issue, eating cholesterol wasn't even mentioned.

And with good reason, in the opinion of Dr. Emil Ginter of the Institute of Human Nutrition in Bratislava, Czechoslovakia. Because the reason why you accumulate cholesterol in your bloodstream and your liver is that you are low on vitamin C. Without adequate ascorbic acid, Dr. Ginter's studies indicate, the body cannot cope too well with surplus cholesterol. And according to Dr. Bernard Caffrey of Clemson University in South Carolina, cholesterol-rich foods like eggs are important because cholesterol plays an important part in the early development of the central nervous system. In Dr. Caffrey's tests with laboratory rats, those fed with high-cholesterol foods like eggs survived emotional stress situations with far greater aplomb than did those on a diet low in cholesterol-containing food.

The textbook *Modern Nutrition in Health and Disease* points out, too, that cholesterol circulating in the blood is not eaten but is manufactured. About 25 percent of the cholesterol in our blood comes from the diet, and 75 percent is manufactured.

"We could cut out all the cholesterol in our diets, and our bodies would manufacture more," says *Prevention* magazine (August 1973).

And according to Professor Mark Altschule of Harvard Medical School, writing in *Executive Health,* "Any real proof of a relation between cholesterol fat and dietary control on the one hand and blood cholesterol levels and heart disease on the other has yet to be established . . . the widespread fear of the cholesterol in food is uncalled for . . . especially regarding our much maligned friend, your morning egg."

And Dr. John Yudkin, professor of nutrition at the University of London, who has concluded a four-year study of the problem, says there is no evidence to relate the number of eggs people eat with the risk of heart disease.

You will probably worry a lot less about the cholesterol in your preworkout morning eggs, however, if you're taking extra lecithin, which is one of those potent plaque-preventing nutrients of which Richard Passwater speaks.

Lecithin, which is known biochemically as "Phosphatidylinositol," is an essential nutrient with important functions in the liver, even if it doesn't trip easily off the tongue.

What is lecithin's special importance to the athlete?

"Lecithin works by improving the circulation," says Dr. Kurt Donsbach. "You can actually see a pale pasty complexion become pink and rosy after using lecithin for a while. Lecithin breaks down cholesterol into tiny bits," says Donsbach. "It does things for your body that nothing else can do. ..." Like strengthening your nerve tissues, improving your tolerance to aspirin, neutralizing numerous poisons, and even increasing brain power and normalizing weight. The word is derived from the Greek word for "egg yolk," which is whence lecithin first came. Nowadays it is extracted from soybeans, and although it is available in a number of different formats, your best bet economically and nutritionally is probably the granular form, which is virtually oil free and 40–50 percent more concentrated than liquid lecithin.

Although its acids contain fat, these fatty acids still have the ability to emulsify fat in foods and in the body. Indeed, as a food, lecithin is a potent emulsifying agent, and once into the body tissues, it assists in the process of fat absorption during digestion, and without fat like this you'll never return to your former thin form.

A tablespoon twice a day of lecithin becomes a superior digestive aid when coupled with your daily dose of vitamins A, D, and/or E. Lecithin is highly perishable like wheat germ and ground nuts and should be refrigerated in a light-resistant container.

Unlike liver and yeast, a taste for lecithin doesn't have to be wincingly acquired. It has a faintly moist nutty flavor that is compatible with virtually anything, which means add it to your dessert, eggs, gravies, soups, and cereals. Lecithin is rich in all the energizing B vitamins but especially in inositol and choline, those two members of the B family on which the health and well-being of your liver is so dependent. Dietarily speaking, all seed foods contain lecithin, but your very best sources are liver, wheat germ, eggs, and unrefined unhydrogenated oils.

Fruits

And now, in our consideration of foods for fitness, we come to the fruits and vegetables and their juices, which keep you in playing if not fighting trim.

According to a report from UNESCO, there is only one people left on the earth who are cancer free. Their diet according to Dr. Ronald E. Gots, "is well-stocked with . . . fresh fruits, vegetables, nuts and grains. . . ."

These disease-resistant people are the by now fabled Pakistani Hunzas, who live at high altitudes in the Karakoram Range of the Himalayas. Not only are they fit as fiddles and presumably still ready for love, but many of them are well over 100!

Super sport Bruce Jenner and his wife share a Hunza like attitude toward the fresh produce in a diet. Says Chrystie Jenner, "One of the things I do in our home is keep a basket of fruit right inside the door of the kitchen. Apples, oranges, and bananas (which contain potassium for strong muscles) are all included, as well as granola snacks and raisins for munching."

Raisins, like all dried fruits, are high-caliber high-octane munching. (Although on the list of the thirty-five foods eaten often by most Americans they place a woeful thirty-one.) Not only are they good candy and snack substitutes, they are formidable repositories of all the major muscle-related minerals and energizing vitamins.

Which fruits have the most magical properties as foods for fitness? Well, there's the avocado, which you should know about if you're a sweathog because it provides more energy per pound than almost any other food. It is as digestible as raw milk and supplies vitamins A, B, C, D, E and K, plus seventeen oils. It is especially high in iron.

And then there is that standard of the breakfast menu, the commonplace orange. It's fine, but the orange is not the only orange fruit with a lot of promise. Consider the apricot. "Together with dried cereals and mulberries, apricots remain a staple food in Hunza," reports the *National Geographic.*

Often called the fruit of paradise, it is one of the most energizing elements in the diet of the fabled Hunzas. According to Rene Taylor, author of *Hunza Health Secrets,* "Scientists have found apricot oil rich in poly-unsaturated fatty acids.... They are a rich source of organic copper and iron which may well be the reason for the absence of anemia in the Hunza people."

Hunzakuts believe that apricots promote their longevity, something nobody says about the orange.

According to *Prevention* magazine, "There is no fruit as nourishing as the apricot, and when they are dried and the moisture removed the nutrients are even greater. They contain large amounts of iron and potassium, and twice the recommended daily allowance of vitamin A."

Nor is the lemon any lemon in this department. It is certainly a central part of what is sometimes called the yoga diet, which many athletes—cyclist and former *Bike World* editor George Beihorn among them—take along with honey before breakfast as an energy booster.

According to nutritionist William R. Dobson, "Citrus fruits contain vitamin A in its provitamin state, and a very good though small amount of the B complex. In citrus have been found eleven amino acids, seventeen carotenoid pigments or provitamin substances and twelve or more bioflavonoids." [6]

Dobson adds that "lemons and oranges alkalinize the system, furnishing useable, well-assimilated calcium and other minerals and making the calcium in other foods available to the cells of the body. They also flush the gall bladder and work as a diuretic; it is really life to the whole body."

An even more popular fruit for sports is the banana.

The banana has been tops among fruits for eleven out of the last twelve years. Ninety-eight percent of American families buy bananas, and last year each family consumed an average of nineteen pounds.

But if you go bananas, do it at the right moment. When unripened, bananas contain only 2 percent sugar. At their peak, they are 18 percent richer in natural fruit sugar.

According to a *Bike World* magazine survey, sixty of the top U.S. racing cyclists said that it was the food they most often ate during races. Maybe it's just because they taste good, but they are a truly superior source of potassium and contain lots of natural carbohydrate, too.

Vegetable and fruit juices are commonly extolled if you run, jump, dive, or otherwise exercise your prerogatives in the right sporting circles.

Juices are uplifting foods in liquid form, as fast-acting as sugar but with none of sugar's drawbacks.

Says N. W. Walker,

Vegetable juices are the builders and regenerators of the body. They contain all the amino acids, minerals, salts, enzymes and vitamins needed by the human body, provided they are used fresh, raw and without preservatives. Whereas, ... fruit juices are the cleansers of the human system but the fruit should be ripe.... Fruits in sufficient variety will furnish the body with all the carbohydrates and sugar it needs. . . .

The addition of one pint of vegetable or fruit juice to the daily diet is one of the greatest safeguards against premature aging and sickness, says Gaylord Hauser.

There is no loss of minerals, vitamins or other nutrients due to overcooking; greater quantities can be taken in liquid than in solid form, and for the aging athlete whose metabolism has begun to slow, juices are a boon.

What makes the juice of vegetables and fruits foods for fitness? What edge does the juice have over the pulp? If it indeed does?

Solid food takes hours of digestive activity to get into the system before its nourishment becomes available to the cells and body tissues. By removing the fibrous matter in your raw fruits and veggies (but not discarding them— that would be throwing away valuable natural food fiber, the stuff that acts as an intestinal broom), the goodnesses of the raw enzyme-rich foods can be instantly taken up by the bloodstream. It is play rather than work, in other words, for your digestive machinery, at a time when you are exerting yourself or are about to. Celery juice, for instance, has a high sodium content and is one of the best drinks to counteract the effects of extreme heat. In contrast, by the time you chomped your way through enough celery to get that special "sweat debt" relief, you'd be too full of roughage to run, with a couple hours' wait for the benefits to start filtering in.

Vegetables

Vegetables for sport? You may have hoped for green beans, but the top honors go to garlic, with onions and radishes a close second.

Actually, garlic isn't a vegetable but an herb. But whatever its classification, it is a small wonder. It energizes, it oxygenates, it keeps cholesterol down and blood sugar up. According to Dr. Paavo Airola, "Garlic and onions are probably the most important health foods of all." Among their other benefits, these two plants seem to have the ability to regulate blood-sugar levels, which is why holistic physicians insist they be liberally used with any hypoglycemic food plan.

According to *Nutrition Reviews,* garlic and onions have demonstrated the ability to prevent increased cholesterol build-up in the blood. Eating large amounts of the two foods has a beneficial effect on blood circulation, too. Reports published in the *Indian Journal of Medicine* showed that blood circulation negatively affected by a high-fat intake could be improved by adding slightly more than 50 grams of onions to the diet—hardly enough to make you shed a tear. What are the properties that produce these near-magical preventive and restorative changes? A substance located in the oils of these vegetables called sulfides.

Roman soldiers reportedly ate garlic before going to battle in the belief that it gave them extra "go" power.

Well, maybe it did. Garlic is 5.3 percent protein, 29 percent carbohydrate, is high in potassium sulphur and phosphorus, and has 1.4 mg. iron for every 100 grams of raw garlic bulb.

Studies by electrobiologist Professor Gurwitch show that garlic stimulates cell growth and has a rejuvenating effect on all body functions. Finnish Nobel Prize winner Dr. A. I. Virtanen claims to have discovered fourteen new beneficial substances in garlic's sister vegetable: the onion. In the USSR, where garlic is referred to as "Russian penicillin," it is used extensively and routinely in hospitals, mostly in the form of vaporized extracts to treat everything from common head colds to uncommon cancers.

Garlic has played a role in reversing atherosclerosis. Dr. Jacobus Rinse, the inventor of the Rinse Breakfast, found that garlic was the only thing that exerted a favorable influence on the course of his atherosclerosis. Dr. Rinse credited garlic with opening up his constricted blood vessels and giving the heart an assist because of its sulphur content, which has antioxidant qualities.

Garlic may well perform its greatest service as a oxygenator of the blood at least this is how Dr. Otto Warburg sees it. In his Noble Prize address, he suggested that where blocked oxidation was a problem, garlic can play an important remedial role. It is an opinion with roots in the past, since garlic has been used since ancient times to help athletes dispel fatigue or boost low oxygen reserves. The prophet Mohammad used garlic, and so does the present-day Mohammad Ali. So it must be the greatest.

Try it next time you have an attack of midgame indigestion. Garlic's even good for that.

Garlic has the added advantage as an herb of being able to pinch-hit for salt, so you can substitute garlic powder or flakes wherever the recipe calls for salt. Anywhere garlic isn't appropriate, kelp (a seaweed) powder will be. Like kelp, garlic is rich in natural iodine, which is easily metabolized by the body.

Will garlic improve your game of tennis? Perhaps not directly, but it may prevent a few of the colds and dyspeptic attacks that kept you off the court, course, or track to begin with. Try some. You've got nothing to lose but a few friends.

What other greens should you eat to stay in the pink? All alkaline-forming plants, such as alfalfa and the leafy greens, are valuable because they neutralize the acid-forming foods and maintain the proper acid-alkaline balance in the body. Spinach, for instance, supplies at least thirty minerals and trace minerals, according to *Environmental Engineering News*.

To put a little extra pow on Popeye's favorite green, you might consider a bit of powdered chili pepper. Chili peppers, says Dr. Lora M. Shields of New Mexico Highlands University, apparently have the ability to lower blood fat levels and reduce the chances of heart attacks.

Persons who eat chili-rich Mexican foods have a longer blood coagulation time, which might spell the difference between health and the occurrence of a stroke or heart attack. Besides, chilis are phenomenally rich in vitamin A. An average serving of some Mexican dishes supplies well over 100,000 units of this vitamin. Chili peppers can also keep good foods from going bad because they act as antioxidants, says a report from the New Mexico State University at Las Cruces.

And then there are soybeans, the kingpin beans of the legume world. They are 2 percent starch and richer in potassium that any other food with the exception of nutritional yeast, which is probably why they have a documented reputation as an antifatigue food. Soybean milk made from dried beans or prepared powder has fifteen times as much iron, no cholesterol, 24 percent less fat, 12 percent fewer calories, 16 percent less carbohydrate, and only one-tenth the amounts of dangerous agricultural chemicals (including DDT) found in dairy milk.

They are also a good source of easily digested energizing vegetable oil. They do, however, yield high levels of copper, which tend to interfere with your dietary intake of zinc, so a diet high in soy products should be supplemented with zinc to be on the safe side. You can add soy to your diet in the form of soy flour, soy flakes, soy milk (now available ready-made), soy grits, and granules (for beefing up meat loaves and baked goods) and as dried, fresh, cooked, and canned soybeans. Or you can eat soybean by-products such as tofu (soy cheese).

Other beans have other virtues. Chickpeas contain twice

as much protein as wheat, and like lentils they are high in all the electrolytes—potassium, calcium, phosphorus, and magnesium—as well as giving you five times the B_2 and ten times the B_1 of most cereal grains.

Grains

Grains and legumes in combination are the classic feel-good food, improved only by sprouting the grain or the bean to add mega-amounts of vitamins and minerals.

And then there are grains, those autocrats of the breakfast training table.

All people known for their superior health and longevity (the Russians, Abhkasians, Hunzas, Bulgarians, Yucatan Indians, for example) make grains the staple of their diet.

However, grains, unlike nuts, should not be eaten raw. The best way to get their maximum value is to sprout them or utilize this nearly cookless cooking method: Bring premeasured grains and water nearly to a boil; clap on the lid and put the covered pot in a 200-degree oven for three to four hours. Neither the proteins, oils, or minerals are damaged or denatured in this way.

Alternately, when time doesn't allow for such long-range preparation, bring the pot to a boil and simmer gently for five to fifteen minutes. Any nutrients that have been damaged may be replaced by tossing in a handful of the same grain, sprouted and minced, or by adding a few teaspoons of nutritional yeast, protein powder or rice polish.

Nonbreakfast eaters are not necessarily excluded from such superbowls. Most cooked grains are just as tasty when appropriately reseasoned as luncheon or supper "mushes," casseroles, etc.

Research supports the idea that grains tend also to be high in the kinds of nutrients that spare the athlete from arthritis, heart attacks, and similar debilitating diseases.

Says Thomas Bassler: "Tissues high in silicon are seen in people who have less arthritis and heart attacks. Foods rich in silicon include rice straw, bran alfalfa (all herb teas), plus pectin plus the hulls of grains (available as 'raw bran' or food fiber)."

And a Czech scientist named Bernasek, who divided rats into two groups, one fed with and one fed without whole grains, found that pathological changes that appeared in the first generation of animals and increased to an acute state in proceeding generations, eventually causing death, were entirely prevented in the group nourished with whole grains.

Unfortunately, however, a kernel of wheat has two sides. "Wheat digestion," say the editors of *Food for Fitness,* "breaking down the dual elements of starch and proteins, demands a certain kind of enzyme production by the stomach, and some of us just don't have the stomach for it. And wheat is one of the major allergens."

So if you are experiencing fatigue (to name only one of a number of symptoms induced by wheat allergy), your diet, rich in homemade bread and whole-grain cereals, may be the culprit.

This unfortunately does not enter into the considerations of some physicians. One of Dr. Robert Atkins' superenergy diets is based on grains, with no warning that it is harmful to some. But you can do without wheat just as you can do without meat.

Buckwheat is an even better bet than wheat. It is less acid forming than wheat, oats, or rye, has less carbohydrate than wheat, and is one of the few crops not doused routinely with chemicals. It is a good source of protein (11–15 percent) and comes closer than any other grain to meat protein. The darker the flour, the more nutritious it is. It's richer in fiber than any other flour, too, and adds no salt to the diet but is a good potassium source. And try one of the less-celebrated cereal grains, millet. Probably the least allergy provoking of all the grains, it is low in sodium, high in potassium, and rich in B vitamins, like all whole grains.

And common folklore to the contrary, it is not rice but millet that is the chief food of the people of north China, where the millet eaters are taller and stronger than their rice-eating neighbors. Why? Because millet is, as tests have demonstrated, the only grain able to support the life of test animals with all the essential amino acids and vitamins when it is fed as an exclusive food. Millet contains lecithin, high amounts of calcium, and is one of the richest sources of B_{17} after sprouts. Millet has the ability to pick up important trace minerals from the soil when they are present there. And it is one of the few grains recommended for low-blood-sugar dieters.

Grains to explore and experiment with include barley, triticale, rye, and rice.

Nuts and Seeds

And then there are nuts and seeds—common peanuts, for instance, which are not nuts at all but legumes, like soybeans. Are they a "shuck" or serious food to train on?

Although no athlete, weekend or otherwise, wants to play for peanuts, they certainly are among the most valuable of fitness foods. As a matter of fact, peanuts are a superior source of the essential electrolyte, magnesium, providing 206 mg. of this mineral, on which so much muscle efficiency is dependent, as opposed to the scanty 28 mg. available in a slice of roast beef.

And peanuts figure in the diets of fit people who have fewer heart attacks as a group. The tissues of such individuals, says runner-writer Thomas Bassler, M.D., are usually high in linoleic acid. "Therefore," suggests Bassler, "eat a lot of peanut butter, wheat germ oil, vitamin E, etc., to keep your tissues full of the 18.2 fatty acid."

In the opinion of nutrition reporter Martin Seifert,

"They are an exceptional food, very rich in the essential amino acids. One whole peanut is equal to 1 gram of peanut-rich oil that in turn is rich in unsaturated fats." But even more amazing to those who have looked into this nut-cum-legume, the peanut both cures and prevents hemophilia, the bleeder's disorder. According to research carried out by Dr. Bruce Boudreaux at Louisiana State University, peanuts actually strengthen the small blood vessels. Other scientific papers report that peanuts have the proven ability to reduce the body's vulnerability to infection and improve the whole efficiency of the cardiovascular system.[7]

Peanuts in particular are plentifully endowed with B_6, pantothenic acid and biotin. The first two are of special value to athletes. And peanut flour is an excellent high-protein ingredient for homemade breads and cereals.

But then all nuts and seeds are veritable pipsqueaks of power, with the highest protein of all found in raw pistachios, so they are especially important in any diet that excludes meat.

Nuts replace meat neatly in mock burgers and loaves and substitute for salty snacks and even for desserts. As Mrs. Janice Stetina, mother of two champion cyclists, says, "There were no gooey desserts around the Olympic village. The Russian athletes thrive on sunflower seeds, and they seem to be way ahead of us in that department."

You should include the super seeds, too, if you're going to be an all-out nut-nut. That means sunflower seeds, which like all seeds and nuts are superior sources of the electrolyte minerals, magnesium and potassium, the ones most liberally sweated away out there on the playing fields. "These little kernels," says *Organic Gardening and Farming Magazine,* "contain practically the whole spectrum of important nutritive elements . . . and almost every vitamin on the chart except Vitamin C. They even develop this one when you sprout them. . . ."

Another top-seeded seed is the lesser known chia seed, something to add to your list of food fuses. It is a form of sage, a member of the mint family and most closely resembles the poppy seed. It is less tasty than most other seeds (its flavor is on the bland side), but its ability to energize the eater is legendary. It once was an important staple in the diet of the Indians of Southern California and Mexico.

The chia is famous for its ability to produce remarkable powers of endurance. Certainly it's worth a try if ever you're feeling a bit seedy.

And when turning to seeds and nuts to bolster your energy stocks, always eat them raw. Cooking destroys 30 percent of the nutrients.

Nuts are best purchased and stored in the shell because this covering protects them from rapid spoilage.

Because they contain so much oil, there is the danger of their becoming rancid. For this reason, it's best not to buy broken or damaged seeds. Oil that has oxidated produces chemical substances that irritate the lining of the stomach, retards the action of the pancreatic enzymes, and destroys large quantities of fat-soluble vitamins. You'll never feel your oats if you're tanked up on spoiled oil.

Nuts in the shell usually stay good for up to a year. Sesame seeds, however, even under the best of conditions, can go bad in six months or less, although sesame oil is the most stable of all the natural oils. One of the best "keeping" methods is to freeze your hulled nuts and seeds and thaw only what you need.

No discussion of nuts and seeds is complete without an examination of the oils extracted from them (as well as the oils extracted from other plants like the soybean and the safflower). And no waters are more troubled than these. Do they lubricate your gears, or just gum up your works?

Polyunsaturated oils, say many experts, perform many jobs in the athletic body. Besides acting as a shuttle system for the fat-soluble vitamins you take in, oils are rich in the kind of fats that keep you feeling well fed and prevent you from getting fat. Any rundown of foods that keep you from feeling run down should include a good oil. But that still leaves a lot of margin for error.

Hydrogenated oils and the foods containing them are the first mistake. Such oils are refined, bleached, deodorized, and emulsified, thereby altering their molecular structure. Both vitamins E and A are destroyed by this processing. They may, in addition, contain propyl gallate, methyl silicone, citric acid, and/or worse.

The desirable fatty acids in them are changed into less desirable ones that your body does not know how to utilize.

Nor should you make a place in your diet for margarine of any race, creed, color, or polyunsaturation. Why?

The toxicity of margarine is due to the fact that hydrogenated oils melt at 114° F or higher, and so enter the blood stream in the form of hard, discrete particles that can clog the capillaries. Nonhydrogenated oils, such as are found in good-quality butter, melt at temperatures far below that of the blood and circulate as a liquid and so do not clog the small blood vessels. Hardened margarine-type oils are found in a wide variety of bakery products, commercial ice cream and junk foods.

If you are on the muscle, you need sound nerves, and polyunsaturated oils have always been considered nerve juice by those in the know. But many authorities disagree. For instance, if there is insufficient calcium in your system to release the benefits of oil's linolenic acids into your blood stream, you may as well be swallowing turpentine.

There are even a few medical practitioners who think you might as well be swallowing turpentine anyway. In their eyes, it would probably be less toxic to you than *any* kind of polyunsaturated oil.

According to one of the pioneers of preventative

medicine, Dr. W. D. Currier, founder of the Academy of Metabology and a member of the International College of Applied Nutrition, "Polyunsaturated oils lower cholesterol by driving it into the blood vessels. You'll get more hardening of the arteries with unsaturated fats than with saturated animal fats."

Currier is not alone in regarding oils as no-nos despite the general impression you may have that oils are unquestionably health promoting and essential tools in controlling cholesterol levels.

Nathan Pritikin, for instance, bans even polyunsaturated fats in his Reversal Diet. He reasons, like Currier, that while these oils may lower the cholesterol level in the blood, not all of the fat actually leaves the body but shifts to the tissues and infiltrates other parts of the body instead.

Says Dr. James M. Iacono, chief of lipid research at the USDA, "At best, the most that man can reduce blood cholesterol by the high intake of polyunsaturated fatty acids is 10 percent."

According to Richard Passwater, you should exercise moderation in using PUFA (polyunsaturated fatty acids) since laboratory rats on diets high in the food element quite readily develop cancer and other diseases. He says, "I have long been aware of the acceleration of the aging process caused by PUFA. ... I find the heavy promo of PUFA dangerous. . . ." [8]

Passwater advises that rather than eliminate saturated fats from your diet, you take in a corresponding amount of unsaturated fats to help the body handle animal products like butter.

Most nutritionists in addition suggest that you look for oils that are labeled cold pressed, meaning fewer of the nutrients, especially the vitamin E, have been destroyed through processing. Or does it mean that?

"Oils labeled cold-pressed may be heated as high as

475° and have other unsatisfactory features about their production," says nutrition reporter Gordon L'Allemand.[9]

Why shouldn't you buy the cheaper, noncold pressed oils in the supermarket? Because "No No. 1-quality peanuts get into an edible oil mill," reporter L'Allemand states flatly. A vast amount of the grain materials from which edible oils are produced is moldy, rancid, stale, bug-contaminated and rat-dung infested." The top-quality peanuts are sold as such for use in candies, peanut butter, or roasted nuts. The spoiled peanut crop is sold at a lower price for oil-making because it has always been the custom of commercial oil producers to refine, deodorize, and bleach their oils.

Rancid oils, remember, are toxic, according to Oberling's *Riddle of Cancer,* Yale University Press. And once rancid, they are beyond redemption.

According to oil expert Frank Lachle, the best way of protecting oil from rancidity is to prick vitamin E capsules and squeeze the 600 IU contents into the quart bottle of oil as soon as it's opened. Shake well and keep refrigerated. Also, keep it in a can or dark bottle.

And if you are using polyunsaturated fats, don't use them in cooking. Once heated, they become resaturated, thereby defeating the purpose for which they are being used to begin with. The degree of saturation becomes worse, says author-internist Edward Pinckney, [10] if the fat or oil is reused (a common custom, especially in restaurants).

Is there any oil that has no unsatisfactory features about its production and about its final appearance?

About the closest thing to the ideal would be Carothers olive oil, the only raw green olive oil around.* It is hand pressed in Europe, not extracted by machine. It is from the

* *Note:* However, olive oil (and peanut oil) are monosaturated oils. They do not have the cholesterol-lowering powers that the polyunsaturated types purportedly do.

first pressing, is rich in natural chlorophyll, and is sealed in cans to prevent destruction of the chlorophyll by light. It is neither heated nor pasteurized. It comes from only the freshest olives. So does a domestic brand called Golden Eagle. It's unheated, untreated, and cold pressed. But of course neither is cheap or easily come by.

Or can't you do what serious raw food vegetarians do for oil? Author Karen Cross Whyte's solution.[11] "One source of raw oil is found floating on top of raw nut and seed butters," she says. "You can skim small amounts of pure oil from the top of the butter as you would get cream from a bottle of raw milk."

And then there are those top-seeded seeds known as sprouts.

"I personally lived on twenty-five cents a day for a whole summer and never felt so good in all my life."

And what could this feel-good-food be that is available for only two bits?

Sprouts. Sprouted vegetables, nuts, and seeds and grains.

"Seeds," continues the redoubtable Ann Wigmore, "are the solution for survival. The stores can close and everything can disappear, but you can still live on sprouts and greens." Miss Wigmore ought to know. She's been touting sprouts for over twenty-five years, is one of the pioneers of raw-food vegetarianism, and runs the Boston-based Hippocrates Health Institute.

If anything is a hedge against the kind of poor diet that eventually does damage to the enzyme systems of the body and the energy-producing systems in the cells, it is sprouted food. And if anything is a food for fitness and a fitting food for sport of any sort, sprouted food wins, green thumbs down.

A sprouted seed is to a seed what a butterfly is to a caterpillar. Sprouting improves the quality, quantity, and availability of a seed's protein.

Dr. Paavo Airola, another sprout booster, adds that

sprouting also improves protein quality in another way. The green leaves that result from sprouting often supply the amino acids that are lacking in the unsprouted part of the seed.

Sprouted alfalfa, for instance, is one of the three natural foodstuffs, according to noted biochemist Dr. Benjamin Ershoff, that can block all or nearly all of the symptoms, from psoriasis to outright death, provoked in lab animals to test the effects of stress.

Sprouted foods often contain 150 times more protein than simple kernels of wheat or corn. And studies show sprouting increases vitamin content by 100 to 1,500 percent.[12] In the case of soybean and sunflower seeds, it develops levels of vitamin C that were totally absent in the seed itself.

All grains, seeds, and nuts in their natural state are foods of fitness, but sprouted, they become the foods on which superperformances can be built. Why? Because their enzyme content increases up to five or six times. Germination releases a flood· of enzymes, and those enzymes digest your food, freeing your body's supply of enzymes to do the repair and maintenance jobs they were intended for and thereby reducing stress and giving you greater energy.

Sprouting not only releases enzymes, it destroys the enzyme inhibitors that many seeds and grains contain.

That is important. Grains, for instance, contain phytic acid to which important minerals are bound, and the digestive system cannot break this acid down without help. Sprouting gives the seed forty whacks, as it were, rendering it into something assimilable by the body at last.

Sprouts also contain considerable natural sugar, in the monosaccharide form, putting them in the category of quick-energy foods. Sprout sugars require little digestive breakdown; therefore they enter the blood stream immediately.

So if you want "get up and go," eat something that gets

up and grows. You can sprout any whole unheated, unsprayed seed, bean, or grain, which means your twenty-five-cents-a-day sprouting diet can run the gamut from sprouted corn and peanuts (use the unshelled, unroasted ones) to leafy buckwheat and sunflower greens (on their final day of germination put them in a sunny window and they'll sprout green leaves) to sprouted brown rice and other things equally nice. Although they are better for you raw, many sprouts are twice as tasty lightly toasted, roasted, stir fried, or steamed. Experiment.

For every booster of sprouts as the perfect food, there is an egghead to claim that title for his favorite food. Oddly enough, an egg, viewed biologically, is a seed.

"I believe that a diet containing a large amount of meat and eggs is dangerous to health," says one authority. "Doctors should tell their patients to eat more eggs," counters Dr. George Briggs of the University of California at Berkeley. "An egg contains only 275 mg. of cholesterol, and the average person's body manufactures up to 2,000 mg. per day. There are only 2 grams of saturated fat in an egg. Eating two eggs a day yields less fat than a normal serving of margarine or salad oil."

And even if you are an egg beater, you cannot ignore the fact that inside this food for fitness is a wonder food: lecithin. The word "lecithin," in fact, means "egg yolk," a food which contains more than 6 percent of that substance.

Eggs are also among the richest sources of vitamin E. They contain large amounts of pantothenic acid, the antistress vitamin.

But there are those who feel you should do without them. Eggs are a no-no in the diet of natural hygienist Aer Waerland, and some natural foodists contend that eggs provide a culture medium, just like meat and fish, for putrefactive bacteria. Others, including Sweden's Professor Kvanda, object to the siderophilic properties of eggs, which result in a binding of dietary iron in the system, much as the phytates in wheat and the oxalates in certain vegetables do.

And those who believe you are what you eat and will play accordingly may not be tempted by the products of a creature who never sees the light of day and lives a short, miserable life on chemically treated mash, which is the fate of most chickens these days.

Wonder Foods

Everybody, no matter what his sport, needs a secret weapon he can sink his teeth into.

There are a number of wonder foods that fit that description. Of course, what lights a fire under Chris Evert may be a fizzle for you, but such is the nature of biochemical individuality. However, in the general arsenal of eating-to-win tools, weapon number one might be:

BREWER'S YEAST: (Also food or nutritional yeast)

"In my list of essentials in life I rank air, water, food, yeast and ascorbic acid. If need be, I would sleep on the streets in a blanket roll if I had to choose between adequate shelter and yeast."

So says H. L. Newbold, M.D., author of *Mega-nutrients*.[13] And if any food is full of meganutrients, it is certainly yeast.

"Brewer's yeast," Dr. William J. Goldswag wrote in *Bestways* magazine, "is about the most potent source of B-complex vitamins that exists in nature. It has the additional advantage of being a live food."

It is also a very old food, going back to the sixteenth century when medical documents indicate it was used as a cure for constipation.

Yeast is a live food, a raw protein, and the smallest plant cultivated by man. It contains all the elements of the B vitamin complex and all the essential amino acids—

sixteen out of the twenty. Just make sure that B_{12} and calcium have been added to the type you buy because it lacks these.

Of the many food yeasts available, brewer's yeast is the best known. As the name implies, it is the spent yeast left after the brewing process. It is cleaned, processed, pulverized, and formulated into tablets, flakes, or powder, usually without the addition of flavorings, preservatives, or additives of any kind.

Nonbrewer's-type yeasts, also called food or nutritional yeasts, are grown solely for use as food supplements, and nurtured on various feeds in large vats until they have produced the maximum number of yeast cells possible. They are then separated from the growing medium, dried at a temperature that is not nutritionally destructive, then through a special process, even the absolute exact mineral and vitamin content can be controlled.

A first-rate source of iron in its natural form, plus eighteen other minerals and micronutrients, it is low in calories, carbohydrates, and costs less than liverwurst. It is also a rich source of antiaging nucleic acids.

Yeast is a concentrated food with a protein content as low as 40 percent, as high as 90 percent. It has virtually no carbohydrate and only about 25 calories in a teaspoon.

Now for the fine points. Picking a yeast is like finding the right tennis racket. It helps to know your species when shopping for a yeast. The name *Saccharomyces cerevisiae* indicates that the yeast has been bred on a solution of purified molasses. (That's good, molasses being a mineral- and vitamin-rich medium.) *Saccharomyces fragilia* means the yeast has been nurtured on whey, the liquid run-off from cheese making, but it may be lower in vitamin-mineral potency than the others. A third strain, *Candida utilis* or *Torula* yeast, is grown on the liquor made from wood pulp.

Brewer's yeast (ñot *Torula*) contains Factor 3, a complex

containing selenium, which augments the action of vitamin E.

New-wave nutritionists like Paavo Airola opt for genuine brewer's yeast, although it has a lower protein content, because it is the best natural source of two very important trace minerals: selenium and chromium. Other yeasts either lack these or supply them in low doses. *Torula* yeast, for instance, according to expert Walter Mertz, is an exceptionally poor source of chromium. Selenium spares vitamin E, increases the body's defenses against stress, improves cardiac function, and more, but who could ask for anything more?

Chromium, on the other hand, is essential for proper insulin function, which is why a deficiency of this mineral often paves the way for diabetes or hypoglycemia. Chromium is essential in the synthesis of many enzymes and hormones and of heart tissue protein. It also plays a part in cholesterol metabolism.

Insulin is the key factor in how the body handles sugar. Dr. A. Mertz of the Nutrition Institute of the USDA says: "The American public gets very little chromium in its food. And the American diet could be providing at least ten times more biologically valuable chromium than it does now." If we all ate yeast, it would.

Nutritionists like Linda Clark and the late Adelle Davis opt for Red Star Yeast, a pure strain of *Ceres Saccharomyces,* because of the sanitary conditions under which it is grown and the good flavor and nutritional potency it delivers.

But all yeasts have rejuvenative properties. In Dr. Clive McKay's study, the addition of only 5 percent yeast to the diet of rats greatly extended their life span maybe because yeast is 15 percent nucleic acid.[14]

If the not-too-appealing flavor of yeast is hard to swallow, you might get acquainted via Vimco, a brand made by Randal Products, which is grown on whey plus buttermilk and has a much milder taste than many other yeasts. The price is low, and the analysis nearly equal to that of brewer's yeast.

How does yeast stack up against other foods with which you may be more familiar? In terms of thiamine or B_1, the "energy vitamin," yeast has approximately ten times as much as dried beans do and twenty times more than liver or lean pork.

If youthfulness is an asset in athletics—and who would argue that it is not?—then yeast is your ticket to ride. It is the richest-known food in nucleic acids. A growing number of scientists, including Dr. Benjamin S. Frank, who is best known for his books on antiaging, believe these to be the key to self-renewal on the cellular level, preserving and even restoring youth. The most immediate effect, observed even in dosages as low as 30 mg. of yeast RNA, is an increase in energy and well-being, Dr. Frank reports. And the higher the dosage, the more rapidly these effects were observed.

So how should you work yeast into your sporting life?

1. You can sprinkle it on buttered or peanut-buttered bread.
2. Take it as part of a pick-me-up drink, stirring a teaspoon or two into a citrus juice, tomato juice, or bouillon.
3. If the taste, which is pleasantly peanutty to some, is unpleasantly unpalatable to you, use it as a hidden ingredient in sauces, meat loaves, stews, breads, etc.
4. If you really want to feel like dynamite, combine your daily yeast with equal, or any desired, amounts of dessicated liver powder. Add lecithin and a niacin tablet, or even a bit of ginseng or pollen.
5. Take yeast on an empty stomach or between meals. But no more than 1 tablespoon at a time to avoid the flatulence that often accompanies eating concentrated high-protein foods like yeast.
6. Yeast should be salivated properly. Don't gulp it down. Once stirred into your chosen solution, eat it with a spoon, or rather chew-drink it.

7. If you are over forty you may have problems with hydro-chloric-acid sufficiency, and a tablet or two of HCL, taken as a digestive aid along with water, may be in order when you prepare to take off with yeast.
8. Flakes probably taste better than yeast in any other form, but the powder is the most potent. Tablets are a convenient source when traveling and for those who cannot acclimate themselves to the taste of yeast, but so many are required to produce any beneficial effects, they are a poor choice.

As a bonus, nutritional yeast is dirt cheap and can be stored indefinitely without refrigeration.

GINSENG

Would you take a quarter teaspoon of something everyday if you knew it was guaranteed to stimulate your digestion, your circulation, strengthen your heart, ease you to sleep at night, and overcome the effects of stress. If you knew it had five thousand years of testing by everybody, including the ancient Chinese?

Then you are ready for ginseng, which is in the front ranks of drug-free uppers. According to American naturopath Dr. Frank Vasquez, "Ginseng is an excellent gland food; a rejuvenator with longevity value; it improves your working output; retards mental and physical fatigue; helps relieve leg and back pain, headaches and dizziness." [15]

For the athlete, ginseng's greatest value is as a nonexciting stimulant. It is an adaptogen, not a drug, and as such it normalizes all bodily functions.

Ginseng's impact on energy and endurance is undeniable.

In the land of skis and cheese, for instance, Switzerland's Consultox Laboratories reported that mice souped up on small doses of ginseng and subjected to swimming tests of stamina and endurance increased their time from 34 to 60 percent the second time around. And in rope-climbing tests staged after the ingestion of only mousy amounts of the legendary "root of heaven," the mice moved with a considerable increase in speed and endurance. Herbalists such as Mary Ann P. Chai define an adaptogen as a non-specific, non-toxic regulator which produces a normalizing effect in all physiological functions; increases mental activity and sustains physical and emotional stability under stress.

One of Russia's leading scientists has been in the forefront of the West's increasing interest in ginseng. He is Dr. I. I. Brekham, of the department of the Physiology and Pharmacology of Adaptation, Institute of Marine Biology, Far East Science Centre, USSR Academy of Sciences, in Vladivostok.

In 1975, he wrote,

Daily doses of ginseng for 15 to 45 days increase physical endurance and mental capacity for work. The increase in efficiency was noted not only during the treatment itself, but also for over a month after the end of the treatment. The increase in work capacity was attended by a number of favorable somatic effects and a general improvement in health and spirits."

"Numerous experiments," says Dr. Brekham, "have shown that ginseng preparations increase physical efficiency and prevent overfatigue." [16]

Dr. Brekham classes ginseng as an example of a completely new genre of drugs, which he named adaptogens, agents which increase the body's ability to deal with stress. According to Dr. Brekham's studies, it does three things of paramount importance to anyone in the thick or the thin of athletics: It affects the function of the blood system, increases muscle tone, and stabilizes carbohydrate metabolism. As a result of these and other findings, ginseng is now as much a staple in the diets of

Russian Olympic athletes and cosmonauts as that over-the-counter poison, the candy bar, is in the diet of the American athlete.

You may not look upon a simple afternoon of squash rackets as something comparable to military combat, but the two situations involve large amounts of physical and psychological stress, which can fray nerves, burn up large amounts of stored vitamins, and lead to indigestion unless there is something like ginseng in the biochemical picture to "increase physical efficiency and prevent overfatigue" as Dr. Brekham puts it.

Which type and form of ginseng should you take, and what are you actually taking when you do?

Ginseng contains a series of glycosides, essential oils, a mixture of fatty acids, ginsenin, phytosterin, mucilage resins, enzymes, vitamins, sugars, a small amount of alkaloids of unknown composition, minerals, and silicic acid.

The synergy is complex. Though glycosides are considered the active constituents, there is evidence that the whole root is more active than any of its separate parts.

There are nine different varieties of ginseng. Russia herbologists rate Siberian ginseng, which is twice as costly as other types, as superior to all other roots of the family. And it also reportedly works its wonders faster in liquid form than capsule or powdered form.

You can double your pleasure, double your fun with ginseng if you couple it with two other healthful healing herbs: fo-ti-teng and gotu-kola. According to Frank Vasquez, they are synergistic to ginseng.

Like that other drug-free pepper-upper, pollen, ginseng should be taken in small doses: One-quarter teaspoon in tea or any beverage is enough.

One lifelong user, Toh Sang Moon, press information officer for the Korean Mission to the UN, makes a batch of ginseng tonic this way: Take two white roots (at sixty dollars a pound they are ten times less expensive than the older red roots) and combine them with a handful of dates in a Pyrex coffeepot full of water. (Metals, except for silver, are said to make ginseng toxic.) After bringing the brew to a boil, Moon lets it bubble gently for about two hours until syrupy. Then he stores it in the refrigerator.

Ginseng is likely to keep your energy levels up longer, and for some athletes it even clears up acne, brings down high blood pressure, knocks out the flu.

Reaction time varies widely. You may notice an increased sense of well-being in a few days, a week, a month, maybe even a few months.

Whatever time it takes, it is worth waiting for.

POLLEN

"Pollen," says Dr. Naum Petrowitsch Joirisch of the Department of Physiology at the Far East Academy Institute of the Soviet Academy of Science in Vladivostok, "is a wonderful biological stimulant with high therapeutic value."

Meanwhile, in another part of our planet, "people have been eating bee pollen for hundreds of years," says Dr. Roger Norse, professor of apiculture at Cornell University. "It's a good rich source of protein, but the idea that it's some sort of elixir is humbug."

Humbug or no, according to the *New York Times* [17] Pollen "is the wonder energy supplement and cure-all of the 1970s. Athletes as diverse as Olympic distance runners and pro basketball players are popping tablets of pollen at the rate of 5 or 10 a day."

Specifically, those pollen-popping athletes include:

- The St John's University track team in Queens. Trainer Jack Gimmler was so impressed with his team's performance after four months on pollen that the university has underwritten a year's supply of the stuff for sixty athletes in four different sports.

- Rutgers University track team. After training on bee pollen, they won two cross-country championships, the first such events they'd won in thirty-eight years.
- At Seton Hall in New Jersey, coach Ion Moon's athletes set an indoor track record for the mile relay in Detroit after three months of pollen supplementation.

Other collegiate athletic departments where pollen is being routinely employed include Fairleigh Dickinson University and Oberlin College in Ohio.

In Finland, national running coach Seppo Nuuttila says that pollen supplements have helped Finnish runners score spectacular successes. In 1967, the country had only one runner among the world's top 100. By 1972 they had 39.

Both the Finnish Olympic team (including Lasse Viren, the 5,000 and 10,000 meter gold medal winner) and the British National Team were among the first athletes to experiment with pollen as a eating-to-win tool. But its use hasn't been limited to runners.

If pollen isn't the bee's knees to some observers, it certainly seems to be the stuff of which gay blades are made.

One of the best-kept secrets in Kremlin sporting circles is that its ice hockey team and a number of its Olympic gold medalists have been popping pollen for years, according to reporter Richard Finnis.

Experts like pollen pioneer Costa Carlsson, the inventor of a unique new method of pollen collection, Chauvin, the French physician, and reporter Rose Wiseman argue that pollen contains the richest sources yet discovered of vitamins, minerals, proteins, amino acids, hormones, enzymes, fats. In short, say experts, every chemical substance needed to maintain life is present in pollen. It is virtually a complete food (yet four ounces of this stuff costs less than a large bottle of Coke). How does it work?

In order to have such miraculous powers, your pollen must be bee collected, which occurs only after the bee gathers and enriches it with nectar.

What precisely is this stuff that makes you fly like a butterfly, sting like a bee? It is the male sexual element of seed plants. Pollen grains correspond to sperm cells in animals and humans.

Pollen is a rich, highly concentrated food that so far has defied synthesization. The 15 percent of it that is fat contains lecithin (another wonder worker); more than 25 percent of pollen is first-rate protein, and more than 50 percent is carbohydrate, the good natural kind. And it has profuse amounts of the B vitamins, the energy complex.

According to the late Leo C. Antles, considered the world's foremost authority on the gathering and curing of fruit pollen over the last forty years and the first person to market pollen nationally to fruit growers, "Pollen is the most potent and complete food on earth."

"The miraculous powers of pollen," Antles wrote, "have been recognized by man since early times. Pollen contains steroid hormones in their natural state. Specifically, among its many other superlative substances, pollen is made up of deoxiribosides, sterines and traces of steroid hormones substances." [18]

Pollen's protein, fat, phosphorus, and iron content resemble most closely that of dried kidney beans, dried peas, and lentils, but it is far richer in minerals such as calcium and magnesium. It is also high in riboflavin (B_2).

And of special importance to the vegetarian athlete is that pollen, according to recent research studies in Sweden and Russia, appears to be one of the very rare plant sources of the elusive B_{12} vitamin.

A Russian report published in 1976 Moscow's Nauka

Press said, "Pollen is a perfectly balanced food containing all 22 amino acids, 27 mineral salts, a full range of the known and probably unknown vitamins and numerous enzymes—all in admirable accord with one another." [19]

Pollen eaters say that the good feelings that this wonder food produces are cumulative, much like the effect of ginseng. Regular consumption brings a feeling of harmony and renewed strength. As one no-longer-weak weekend athlete put it: "This regeneration of body practically borders on a miracle." The reason is that pollen possesses what have been described as super detoxicating and constructive properties.

Moreover, pollen seems to offer a hedge against the ravages of stress, according to Dr. Peter Hernuss at the Women's Clinic at the University of Vienna. In laboratory tests, the regular administration of 60 grams daily of pollen to women stricken with radiation sickness boosted their vitamin E levels by 36 percent, lowered cholesterol levels by 14 percent and elevated vitamin C levels 33 percent. Total blood protein also rose by 13 percent.[20]

It even tastes good, and if you've given up those sugary chocolate shots on top of your ice cream, here's a whole new wrinkle in dessert sprinkles to replace them.

Mohammad Ali uses it, and so does gold medalist Steve Riddick. Its history as an athletic booster goes back to the original Olympic athletes, who used bee pollen as part of their food-psyching formula for extra energy.

So can you. At about a buck for 4 ounces—do some comparison shopping before you buy—it's a bargain.

LIVER

Wonder foods like liver are multiple-course meals in themselves. Few foods that look and taste as unpromising as liver does, whether freshly cooked or desiccated (dried) into tablets and powders, deliver anywhere near the total nutrition that it does. "Pound for pound" says the editor of *Lets Live* Magazine (March 1978) "there's no food which contains so many invaluable nutrients as liver ... liver is one of the foods richest in vitamin B-2 (riboflavin) which has been found by various experiments to help develop energy and endurance ... delay old age and senility and build resistance to disease."

Liver provides distinct power to the people who take it to put shots, pop flies, push pedals, or pin their opponents, whatever their game is. It is, of course, a famous source of iron. Bronze medalist runner Kathy Hammond, who generally spurns supplements, admits she takes iron (liver) pills regularly. U.S. weightlifting champ Paul Grippaldi takes liver-protein tablets with every meal.

Even strong-willed vegetarians sometimes sneak liver into their diets, none with a more ingenious rationale than George Bernard Shaw's: "It is my medicine."

Dr. B. H. Ershoff, professor of biochemistry at Loma Linda University School of Medicine, conducted a dramatic test of its power. When generous amounts of dessicated whole liver were added to the diets of stressed test animals fated to die in thirty days of heart failure, they were "totally protected." And when 10 percent of their total diet was replaced by brewer's yeast, they lived five times longer than those without it.

As author Richard Passwater reports, "Experiments have been conducted in which animals given all the known vitamins do not survive long. Other animals similarly treated but also given liver or various liver extracts live normally."

Any athlete trying to push his or her oxygen intake up over seventy (distance runners, for instance) can't afford even a mild case of iron-deficiency anemia. Fortunately, that can be prevented or remedied by adding iron-rich liver to the diet. In tests conducted by Dr. B. H. Ershoff, again reported in the *Journal of Nutrition,* rats were divided into three groups, with only the final group receiving dessicated liver as a portion of their daily diet. At the end of three months, the rats were pitted against one another in a test of swimming endurance, one of the best barometers of stamina. Both of the liver-unfortified groups expired after 13 minutes, while the liver-loving rodents were still in the swim after 120 minutes. Further tests with liver-fed laboratory animals have demonstrated the exceptional energy-producing values of this superfood. Liver is a blood builder, a superior source of iron and all other major minerals, and like yeast, a superior source of every B vitamin.

Liver contains more vitamin A than just about any other food, 45,000 units in one-quarter pound. However, since most of this is contained in the fat of the organ, dessicated liver that is also defatted will deliver a somewhat lower payload of A. Since the iron in liver occurs naturally, many nutritionists feel that we probably absorb it from liver with more efficiency than from other sources.

If you decide to put liver in your diet, you might consider the question of its source. Many liver lovers feel that products processed from Argentine or Canadian cattle are superior because liver from these smog-free areas is also free of insecticide and pesticide contamination.

Next to fresh, lightly cooked liver, dessicated liver that is dried at very low temperatures to retain full nutrient value is the most valuable supplement available for protein, B vitamins, and iron, in the opinion of many nutritionists. Best of all is raw liver powder. Its nutritional value is only minutely less than that of liver in its raw, fresh state because the liver is dried at an even lower temperature.

If you take three tablets (500 mg. each), you get the equivalent of 3 ounces of fresh meat.

WHEAT GERM

You've hardly begun to do any food tripping for the sake of your sport, however, if you haven't taken the heart of the wheat kernel to heart.

For just as wheat germ is separated from the rest of the grain in processing, we now must separate the germ, for purposes of discussing it, from the rest of the grain. The germ is the inner seed of a kernel of wheat, like a seed in fruit. However good the grain itself, it is the germ that most benefits the athlete.

And even here we must further fractionate the germ from its own oil. Wheat-germ oil contains the fat-soluble vitamins, mostly E, but it is not as good a source of the B vitamins or of protein as wheat germ itself.

Wheat germ is among the best-known sources of the minerals selenium, magnesium, manganese, copper, potassium, and phosphorus, the mineral that helps thin the blood of excess fat.

Wheat germ has four times as much protein as an egg, eight times more protein than white bread, and more B_1 than any other food except yeast. Its protein is on a par with soybeans, and since it has a lower nitrogen content than other whole grains, it is easier on the kidneys. It's one of the few protein foods that can be eaten uncooked and should be for the greatest benefit.

Wheat germ is rich in all the B vitamins, but especially pantothenic acid, the antistress vitamin, and B_6, which helps to metabolize protein. Its only failing as a balanced nutrient is its lack of calcium, but if you eat your daily ration swizzled into a cup of yogurt, you're covered.

It is certainly a must for anybody on a losing streak or a high-protein diet, or both. For instance: In a remarkable series of studies in 1956 at the University of Illinois, T. K. Cureton increased the stamina of a group of Olympic swimmers by 51.5 percent simply by adding wheat germ and its oil to their daily fare for period of three months. The wheat-germ-fed swimmers outranked the competition in all events.

Because of its large amounts of vitamins B and E, wheat germ keeps the capillaries of the heart tissues open, increasing the flow of blood in the arteries.

Dr. Cureton's twenty years of research on wheat germ and its oil has been reported on by himself and many others in numerous journals including *Research Quarterly, Scholastic Coach,* and the *Athletic Journal,* as well as in a book published in 1968 by Charles C. Thomas entitled *The Physiological Effect of Exercise Programs on Adults.* Dr. Cureton has worked his wonders with wheat germ on swimmers, runners, and wrestlers. His conclusions are that this wonder food improves endurance and stamina, reduces heart stress, and quickens reaction time.

Swimming coach Dr. Forbes Carlisle reported similar successes with Australian Olympic swimmers prepared six months before competition by a diet fortified with wheat germ, wheat germ oil, and additional vitamins and minerals.

Such supplementation, commented a report in Australia's *Journal of Physical Education,* "Was an important factor in maintaining endurance during the 1960 Olympics."

But a few guidelines before you begin sprinkling and swallowing: Wheat germ oil works best in partnership with exercise, just the way wheat germ is potentiated when it is coupled with ascorbic acid. There is a synergy in both cases that stimulates the production of muscle glycogen.

In some of the Cureton experiments, it was shown that wheat germ, taken daily after exercise by active subjects, produced greater results than when taken by sedentary subjects.

Wheat-germ oil capsules are an excellent supplement, according to Dr. Harold Rosenberg, a vitamin therapist, if they are fresh. Unfortunately, he notes, "All natural vegetable oils including wheat germ are highly reactive and can readily become rancid, losing up to 40% of their nutritional values within a short time." And *Health Survival Digest* adds, "A daily wheat germ supplement is not enough if you're looking for the beneficial therapeutic uses of vitamin E. Even if the germ was only 1 or 2 days old you would need a few ounces of the oil to secure 500-600 units of the active alpha tocopherol."

A good dose schedule to follow might be one teaspoon of oil or 7-10 large capsules before breakfast or before retiring.

This loving spoonful daily, down the hatch or mixed in with your salad oil or anything else that won't be heated, raises the oxygen in the heart and other muscles and the tissues by 30 percent, the equivalent effect of an oxygen tent, according to nutrition reporter Linda Clark.

Russian studies indicate that the nervous system is affected by supplementary feedings of wheat germ oil. And linoleic acid, which is a heart-muscle nutrient, comprises up to 50 percent of wheat germ oil.

If you're playing the percentages, wheat germ oil and/or wheat germ itself are nutrients not to be missed. After all, anything that Gary Player carries around in his back pocket has got to be pretty up-front stuff.

VITAMIN B₁₅

If you'd rather feel boffo than blotto, if indeed you would like to feel the greatest, maybe B_{15} is your superfood. According to Richard Passwater, Mohammad Ali's doctor, during one of the champ's lows,

> Ali's blood was at a low sugar and low iron level. Ironical that the world's heavyweight champion was on the way to weakening iron-deficiency anemia. Because Ali was to fight contender Jimmy Young within the

month, I suggested that he consider taking pangamate (B_{15}), chelated iron, and other supplements for a well-rounded supernutrition program. Within three days, his blood was normal again, and his desire to train returned. . . .

B_{15} so exceeds the bounds of any other do-good vitamin that it is more logically classed with wonder foods than vitamins. It does have, however, in common with the other B vitamins a high safety factor because it too is water soluble.

The American Chemical Society Abstracts indexes it as B_{15}, yet it is not officially recognized as a vitamin by the FDA. Biochemists call it "pangamate." It is a nonfuel nutrient in the diet that has remedial properties. Biochemist Richard Passwater, who considers it as important as Vitamin E, calls it "the oxygen vitamin" or the "blood vitamin."

Why? Because as a team of prominent Russian scientists wrote in the Reports of the Academy of Sciences, USSR, in 1962, "Our results indicate that B_{15} increases general and myocardial resistance to hypoxia," meaning a better supply of oxygen to the heart's muscle tissue.

Pangamate, according to Passwater, also "promotes the building of muscle, increases oxygen transport efficiency within the cell, restores reflex time, increases stamina and wind, removes the sluggishness and inertia that keeps an athlete from aggressive training. It increases his tolerance for hard work."

Most of the findings on B_{15} come to us courtesy of the Russians. For instance: Dr. Yakovlen of Leningrad demonstrated that B_{15} has a positive effect on the metabolism during extensive athletic endeavor, reducing the oxygen debt and oxygen saturation. His colleague, Dr. Leshkovich, demonstrated in 1962 that pangamate was equally helpful during shorter, more intensive bouts of exercise, causing a marked increase in the utilization of fats as an energy source.

The two doctors jointly reported in 1964 that even before these changes took place in the body of the exercising athlete, there was a notable decrease in the formation of lactic acid build-up, which signals the onset of fatigue. There also was a lower output of muscle glycogen reserves and an increase in the levels of muscle creatine-phosphate, plus improved fat metabolism in general. All of this was observed with the administration of only 5 mg. of B_{15}.

Pangamate seems to work best for short-burst energy expenditures, when there is an almost certain disturbance in the energy balance. Its effects are most profoundly felt when taken for three days in succession. Following the last dose, the effect may linger another four days, says Passwater. It is similar in this respect to the way in which the "nucleic acid cure" works, as described by Dr. Hans Kugler. If you are an athlete or near-athlete who has arrived at the watershed years, it is good to know that pangamate also has the power to normalize the ratio of sodium to potassium in the heart muscle, according to research by Dr. Apanasenko of the Medical Institute of Blagoveschensk-On-Amur, USSR, as reported by Dr. Passwater. In addition, it provides the methyl groups needed to detoxify poisons, make lecithin, and help in slowing down the aging process.

Again, according to Passwater,

Athletes—and especially athletes once thought to be past their prime—have benefited greatly from pangamate.

Since it increases the supply of available oxygen, athletes will have greater wind and more reserve.

Other advantages of pangamate to the athlete, old or young, include improved physical energy, less fatigue, increased muscle size and strength and faster healing of injuries.

In addition to all this, B_{15} seems to protect and control more serious disease than any other vitamin and even helps to control a runaway sweet tooth and the craving for junk food by normalizing and regulating blood sugar levels.

Taken as a supplement, it is especially effective in a piggyback combination of B_{15}, A, and E.

Since it is not included in most vitamin formulas, a healthy supply of B_{15} may have to come from B_{15}-rich foods themselves. Topflight sources are pumpkin and sunflower seeds and brewers yeast, whole grains, rice bran and rice polish, and apricot kernels. For tablets, look in your health-food store for the one or two imported brands, from Germany or Russia, now on sale here.

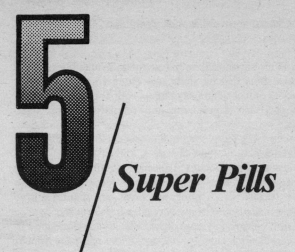

5 / *Super Pills*

Maybe you aren't going for gold medals, but you should know that some vitamins and minerals are veritable silver bullets. And you can psyche yourself upward or down with certain food supplements, just as you can with certain foods.

There are a number of common over-the-counter vitamins and minerals that provide legitimate nontoxic, nonexpensive natural hormonal highs or lows.

As any drugstore nutritionist will tell you, all systems of the body in some way or another rely on the efficient functioning of the nervous system. There are, for instance, six thousand internal adjustments that the body must make regularly that are dependent on a single electrolyte, magnesium.

What other minerals and what vitamins are needed to make overall body functioning efficient?

"Vitamins," says Dr. Richard You, U.S. Olympic Games team physician, "mean the difference between a champion and an also-ran." He adds that most athletes suffer from nutritional deficiencies from time to time.

And further supplement endorsement, admittedly a bit tempered, comes from Dr. Benjamin Frank: "Vitamins help a little but do not in themselves increase energy and athletic performance as strikingly as a nucleic acid-rich diet does, particularly when supplemented with nucleic acid tablets." [1]

"Vitamin balance and physical—especially athletic—performance capacity are closely related. In all clinical cases of vitamin deficiency the first symptom to appear is reduction of physical capacity." So begins a paper by one of Austria's most respected sports physicans, Dr. Ludwig Prokop, discussing individual vitamins and their role in athletics, in the journal *Der Lecihtathlet.*

Endurance capacity is often not so much a question of taking vitamins in high dosages but assuring the simultaneous working of various vitamins in a physiologically balanced bouquet.... This is above all true of A, B_1, B_2, C and E.

In hard work, the need for various vitamins increases markedly so that even with so-called normal doses a deficiency can occur.

For athletes Dr. Prokop has found the daily need to be two to three times higher than normal. He recommends extra amounts of E and C, both specific to endurance and recovery, plus higher levels of almost all the vitamins.

Vitamins do, in general, act as catalysts, speeding up many reactions but not being used up as they do. Vitamins C and E, however, self-destruct in the course of doing their jobs and must be supplied in larger quantities than the others.

Are you getting enough of what you need?

One clue to a vitamin-deficiency state, said Adelle Davis, is an excessive appetite, which "usually indicates an inadequate diet, especially of the B vitamins."

The energy alphabet for any athlete begins with the B complex, especially B_1, B_3, B_6, B_{12} and another so beatific it has been promoted to wonder-foods status (B_{15}).

Dr. Ludwig Prokop calls these the "performance-specific vitamins." Just as B_1 in goodly supply is needed to handle any increase in exercise or endurance performance, B_2 is needed to enhance endurance activity because of its importance in the formation of respiratory enzymes.

Runners' coach Ernst Van Aaken recommends being sure you're getting all of your Bs by taking them in the form of dried nutritional yeast, which contains all thirteen members of the group.

W. D. Currier also opts for B vitamins from food first: "B complex vitamins in natural foods are absorbed many times more efficiently than the same amount in tablet form."

It is important to point out the distinction between the B vitamins and all the other vitamins.

Without elaborate chemical wordfare on the mechanics of vitamin metabolism, B vitamins are water soluble, which means that most people can experiment with them in large, even mega doses without fear of poisoning themselves. Most bodies will discard any amount they cannot use or store.

This is not so with A and D, however. And in the case of vitamin E, it is customary to work up to the higher levels, observing first how the body deals with each level. Some individuals have difficulty tolerating the higher doses. This is also true in the case of niacin (B_3), which must be carefully administered to some diabetics, for example. But these are the exceptions. If you are healthy, you should be able to benefit from rather high doses of vitamin B. Many nutritionists recommend experimenting with the B vitamins one by one to find the level of dosage that lights your fire. What works for your tennis partner won't necessarily work for you. In general, it is important to work out a personal plateau for each B vitamin and then balance them, since the B complex is the body's major energizer among the vitamins.

However big other dietary nutrients may loom in licking athletic lethargy, they are mere pikers compared to the B vitamin complex. You can get a buzz just from taking certain B vitamins. For starters, you might begin at the beginning with B_1, otherwise known as thiamin.

Dr. H. L. Newbold recommends you begin with a 500-mg. capsule after breakfast on a Saturday morning. Why 500? Because less is rarely worthwhile. And on Saturday because it is possible, says Newbold, that "you will experience a high and need some time to come down."

B_1 is celebrated as the "morale" vitamin. It is a necessary part of the body's enzyme system, used in helping the body to distribute and burn sugar to produce energy.

"The athlete," said Adelle Davis, "if he be really first class, must have more than an ample supply of thiamin. The best dancers, distance runners, swimmers, and mountain climbers also need an abundant amount. . . ."

A simple increase in thiamin sometimes doubles the capacity for work without undue tiring.

Thiamin is required in proportion to carbohydrate intake, an important consideration since you will probably be taking in more carbohydrate as your activity levels accelerate. When thiamin is inadequately supplied, the heart is the first organ in the body to suffer. As Adelle Davis put it, "There is no doubt that you who wish to go wondrously through life with strong sound hearts must carefully plan your diets to include generous amounts of thiamin."

How generous an amount and how to include it?

You can wipe out fatigue and depression effectively with 500 to 2,000 mg. daily, says Dr. Robert Atkins.

Meat, brewers yeast, wheat germ, and nuts are good ways to mainline B_1, but for megadoses, use a starch-and-sugar-free capsule of B_1 at whatever potency you feel comfortable with. Bear in mind that a capsule containing the entire B complex should accompany any additional amounts of single B vitamins taken to prevent difficiencies. In general, thiamin intake should be jacked up as you jack up the caloric or carbohydrate content of your diet. It should be kept high to compensate for the B_1 you're missing if your diet is moderately high in processed "junk" foods.

East German swimmers, for instance, are administered half a gram of B_1 as part of a diet that provides 4,000 calories daily. You can even escalate and take 3,000 mg of B_1 (divided into three installments), says Dr. Newbold, if you feel your good feelings soaring and your game improving.

An even better upper, say some nutritionists, including Paavo Airola, is the combination of aged garlic extract, liver extract, and vitamin B_1. It is available commercially, but you could put it together yourself; cured garlic is just mashed raw garlic that's been aged in wood or in a crock for anywhere from thirty days to two years.

But what if you fail to find your "good feelings soaring"? What if you're still in a slump even with all that extra B_1 burbling around inside?

It is probably your "biochemical individuality" that is the culprit. As biochemist Roger J. Williams puts it,

We can list the quantity of a nutrient required by the majority of adults. We could then compile a list of five nutrients, each with the quantity required by the majority of adults. However, few adults would have their needs met with the quantities listed. The data would necessarily only apply to three percent of the adult population.[2]

Assuming that you have no fear of flying, you can proceed to B_3 (niacin). But remember, it is not for diabetics.

One good reason why you need extra B_3 is because it participates in the enzymatic breakdown of sugar at several places in the body's energy cycle. A deficiency of this substance has a marked effect in slowing down brain metabolism, something you can ill afford.

Niacin is indispensable in metabolizing carbohydrates, fats, and protein, and twice the usual dosage may be barely enough if you're active.

B_3 produces a feeling of increased well-being that takes several forms, depending on the particular human system it is shuttling through. Sometimes it produces restlessness, at other times, a good deal of drive or simply a more "alive" sensation. Unfortunately, it has one annoying side effect. It is also accompanied by a "flush" and an itchy tingling sensation that may persist for an hour or longer because niacin releases histamine from the basal cells in the body. Begin with doses no higher than 250 mg.

But that is rather a small price to pay for a nutrient that will prolong your life, reduce your serum cholesterol, increase the oxygen-carrying abilities of your blood, prevent your bloods from clotting too readily, raise your blood-sugar levels, and reduce tension and depression. And put you in the mood to win.

B_3 is also available as niacinamide. This form of B_3 does not produce the flushing and itching of the skin that niacin does, but it doesn't produce the energy "highs," either, and in megadoses may produce depression in certain susceptible individuals.

Another member of the B vitamin complex considered a hedge against energy deflation is folic acid, the foliage vitamin, named for the green spinach leaves that are so rich in it. Actually, it is another one of the dual upper-downer nutrients, since as Dr. Newbold says, "Depending on the individual, megadoses of folic acid may either stimulate or sedate."

Folic acid is one of those last-chance nutrients tried by nutritional therapists when all other attempts to cope with fatigue and sagging energy levels have failed.

"The overwhelming majority of those people for whom vitamin therapy does not seem to work either do not follow a careful enough diet along with their vitamins, or their vitamin regimen does not contain enough folic acid," says superenergy author Dr. Robert C. Atkins. One of the reasons that your diet may be deficient in folic acid is that every step in the processing of food—canning, freezing, heating, pasteurizing, storing, shipping, etc.—wipes out a bit more of this fragile nutrient, so that most processed foods retain no more than 5 percent of the folic acid they started with.

Another reason is that unlike Canada and other countries where you can pop folic acid like salted peanuts if you choose, in the United States you can buy tablets of no more than .4 mg. without a doctor's prescription.

According to one expert, Dr. Victor Herbert, the symptoms of folic-acid deficiency include fatigue, weakness, shortness of breath, symptoms not unlike those of a B_{12} deficiency, with which folic acid should always be taken. Herein lies the reason the government limits the tablet size. Folic acid may mask a B_{12} deficiency with serious results, including irreversible brain damage.

But insufficient folic acid has consequences, too: poor absorption of all that expensive vitamin E you are taking, for example. So maybe it's worth the time and trouble of counting out and tossing off those thirty or more little tablets to get the 10 mg. of folic acid you need daily, but always with B_{12}. Food sources of folic acid include wheat, asparagus, leafy greens, liver, but it's a fair bet that you'll never eat enough organically grown beet greens or fresh liver to get 10 mg. daily.

If you are megadosing with vitamin C, then you are certainly losing a high percentage of folic acid in your urine. Some experts estimate the loss is as high as 75 percent and is pushed even higher if you have absorption problems, intestinal disorders, or are just plain past your prime. This amount may be replaced by supplementation without fear since folic acid is a water-soluble nutrient that the liver stores for short periods. Another folic-acid authority, Kurt A. Oster, chief of cardiology at Bridgeport's Park City Hospital, uses up to 80 mg. a day to combat hardening of the arteries. This is a far cry from the government's recommended dose of .4.

Pantothenic acid is a biochemical precursor of the adrenal hormones and is found in great quantities within the adrenal gland tissues.

The life span of test animals has been extended by feeding them pantothenic acid-rich diets, according to its discoverer, Roger J. Williams. One important source of this vitamin is Royal Jelly—smaller amounts are found in honey, too—which explains the legends about Royal Jelly's rejuvenating powers.

The ratio of pantothenic acid to B_1 in human muscle is 11 to 1, and the ratio in milk and eggs is also a generous 10 to 1. This is twice the amount contained in other animal muscle such as pork, chicken, beef, etc. All of the calcium pantothenate (as it also is known) must be supplied by our diets, a fact that seems lost on vitamin manufacturers, who persist in producing B vitamins and multivitamin supplements with inadequate ratios of these two nutrients. Although pantothenic acid means "from everywhere," the substance is hardly as widespread as many conventional nutritionists would have you believe, since it is readily destroyed by toasting, roasting, and other heat treating.

Large amounts are also destroyed by simple stress, which is of course an inescapable element in athletics no matter how moderate your involvement.

Next to E, the most controversial vitamin for sport is C, or ascorbic acid. As with E, the controversy rages over whether it is even a vitamin. It is really a liver metabolite, insist those who have done the most thoroughgoing studies.

And it is the inability to manufacture any of this metabolite that puts us in the same biochemical boat with the fruit-eating bats of India.

They, like us, cannot synthesize their own ascorbic acid, in contrast with most of the rest of the animal kingdom. Most animals manufacture a certain amount of C for every kilogram of body weight. Extrapolating from this, the human need would work out to approximately 3,830 mg. of ascorbic acid, a figure that is at considerable variance with the government's recommended daily allowance of 45 mg.!

Under stress, moreover, which almost any form of athletics involves, the requirements go much higher. Not only is it virtually impossible to get enough vitamin C into your system by systematically eating all the citrus fruit in sight, but also, in the expert opinion of H. K. Stieberling, the national food supply is 15 percent lower in vitamins A and C than it was twenty years ago.

Whatever it is that's in sixty-seven glasses of fresh orange juice, a day's supply of C if you don't take tablets, you need a lot of it.

A single teaspoon of crystalline powdered vitamin C, the more practical way to get the equivalent of all that liquid sunshine, is a lot more than a contraceptive for the common cold. *Although,* that aspect is nothing to sniff at if you've ever run a road race with the flu.

Fewer colds, of course, mean more days on the court, course, road, or rink for you. For testimony to the fact that most of us are undersupplied with this metabolite, which the bodies of cats and dogs make automatically, compare the number of "dog" days you suffer, compared to those your family dog or cat has, due to colds.

Ascorbic acid also is a Grade A upper.

"Both Mrs. Pauling and I found that we experienced an increased sense of well-being, general aliveness and good health when we increased our intake of Vitamin C," says Linus Pauling, certainly C's biggest booster.

Further, Pauling states that a steady intake of vitamin C from birth might well increase your longevity by twenty-four years.

What if you haven't been getting quite the results you have been expecting with C? Take it with wheat germ and stand by. According to Dr. Szent-Gyorgyi, the biochemist who isolated both vitamin C and vitamin P (the bioflavonoids complex), you can potentiate your body's supply of ascorbic acid by coupling it with fresh, raw wheat germ. A breakfast that does this every day is what has kept the good doctor hale, hearty, and cold-free at the age of eighty.

Two ounces of germ with milk and sliced fruit each day is one way of doing it. Then sprinkle in your powdered C or take the number of tablets required.

Another reason to increase your intake: C is a super-oxygenator, and a fresh slug of oxygen is like the proverbial shot of adrenalin.

"Massive doses of vitamin C injected into the blood stream," says Dr. Fred Klenner, possibly the world's leading authority on this nutrient, "release a tremendous amount of oxygen. And C in the body builds a network of tissue within the bones to hold an extra supply of minerals. Without C, the minerals cannot be deposited, and the bones suffer."

A lack of vitamin C also reduces the body's ability to tolerate carbohydrates, which is not a good state of affairs if as a civilian-athlete you are depending on carbohydrate for energy. Ascorbic acid also helps deposit calcium into bone structure and replaces it when it is needed. And note that if your ascorbic acid levels are at ebb tide, you may get heightened cholesterol levels in your blood because "C" is essential in the process of converting cholesterol into bile.

"Vitamin C undoubtedly occupies a central position in connection with performance ability," says Ludwig Prokop. This substance is partially responsible for the economy of almost all metabolic processes in the body. . . . A deficiency reduces physical-performance capacity, and during physical exertion, the underbalance of it is intensified." [3]

Prokop also considers vitamin P, more commonly known to us as the bioflavonoids, performance-specific, "The vitamin P complex (rutin, citrin, hespirin) used in relatively large amounts by the body has a certain indirect influence on performance because of its stabilizing effects on C as well as possibly other water-soluble vitamins."

At medical gatherings in corners where conservatism still prevails, nobody closes the doors on vitamin C. Dr. A. Venerando, speaking at the International Symposium on the Nutrition of Athletes in Leningrad (1976), reported that ascorbic acid did contribute to alleviation of lactic acidosis associated with athletic energy expenditures, even, he added, if hard evidence that it improved work performance wasn't at hand.

At the Research Center of Metabolism and Nutrition in Prague, however, the evidence seems sufficiently hard to make Czechoslovakian medical workers soft on C. Workers report that vitamin C's effect on flu-infected coal miners was to increase their vigilance. And further studies, says the *Review of Czechoslavakian Medicine,* confirm the evidence that C makes workers more "alert."

Why not? C might well be called the thinking man's

vitamin. There is more C in the brain than anywhere else except the adrenal cortex and it is the brain that directs your feet to do their stuff out there on the playing fields.

How can your feet do their stuff if your tendons and arteries are prematurely aging? This is what happens, says gerontologist Richard Passwater, when tissue levels of C are perilously low. Bring them down even lower and you experience the extreme fatigue that is associated with that vitamin C deficiency state called scurvy.

What kind of C to take, when and how much? And what about natural versus synthetic vitamin C?

Synthetic ascorbic acid is just as effective as natural sources of vitamin C, says Dr. Pauling. On the other hand, according to a report by the Rodale publication, *Organic Gardening and Farming,* one natural source, *Roga Rugosa* (rose hips), contains anywhere from 500 to 6,000 mg of C in 100 grams, in addition to A, B_1, B_2, E, and K. An orange weighing 100 grams has only 50 mg.

There are even further decisions to make when you go comparison shopping for C, natural or otherwise. According to Dr. Richard Passwater, the only form of C that the adrenal cortex will store is calcium ascorbate. So if you aren't taking that, you should be taking calcium and ascorbate together to do the trick. Without this vitamin-mineral fusion, major hormones cannot be produced, says Passwater.

High doses of vitamin C also cause a certain inevitable irritation of the kidneys and the bladder, but this can be buffered somewhat if you are taking in adequate minerals. Otherwise, this diuretic action may also result in a loss of the body's stored minerals. Another consideration in taking megadoses of ascorbate is the amount of sodium you are getting along with the ascorbate. Sodium ascorbate ... taken in non-timed form ... has less diuretic action. However, it contains about 11 percent sodium so most people will prefer to avoid it. ...

One way to arrive at the amount of C which is adequate for you is to measure the amount of stress you're under.

If the stress you're under is definitely more than bush league, you will probably need between 6,000 and 10,000 mg. of C a day. Ascorbic acid certainly won't function as an "upper" at levels lower than this. Dr. Klenner suggests 20 grams, the amount he takes himself.

"There is little doubt," says Dr. Pauling, "that exercise causes an increased requirement for ascorbic acid. Something like six grams a day might be desirable for people who are under stress of one sort or another." (While the nonactive average individual needs four times the Required Daily Minimum, the active adult needs even more.)

The easiest and most economical way of megadosing with ascorbic acid is using its crystalline form (one-quarter teaspoon equals 1 gram) mixed with orange juice. (The juice is there not for its ascorbic acid, but for the bioflavinoids or vitamin P content, nutrients not found in the C powder itself.)

Powdered rosehips is also available. And it doesn't taste bad. Recipes incorporating both forms of C powder are included in the recipe section.

Vitamins B_6 and B_{12}

"Some of the swimmers are pill freaks," said Mark Spitz, "especially (of) B_6 and B_{12}. I think it just gives them a mental lift or a type of placebo power."

Lift or rip-off? What is the real B_6, B_{12} story?

According to *Meganutrients* author Dr. H. L. Newbold, B_6 is one of the most important vitamins, especially for anyone on a high-protein diet, because B_6 is involved in protein metabolism. But it also figures in carbohydrate metabolism, so that any special athletic diet should pay special attention to B_6.

"When you begin taking pyridoxine (B_6)," says Newbold, "you may find that you have more energy, feel less tense, lose any bloated feeling in your body. . . . You may find that it relaxes you to the point of sleepiness. . . ."

Reporter Roseann C. Hirsch calls B_6 the vitamin for nerves and muscles and suggests an extra 5 or 10 mg. daily to anyone who suspects his B vitamin intake may not be quite up to snuff in the pyridoxine department. Dr. Newbold advises 100 mg. three times daily, which is the dosage he takes himself. The government's recommended daily allowance of 2 mg. is considered very skimpy by many nutritionists, and Dr. Carl Pfeiffer of the Brain Bio Center in Princeton, N.J., thinks 25 mg. is far more reasonable.

Acting as a coenzyme, B_6 is responsible for over sixty biochemical reactions in the body, one of which, assisting in the metabolism of carbohydrates, is of special interest to the athlete who is usually a big carbohydrate consumer. B_6 is involved in the health of the entire adrenal cortex, so it is probably important to have large doses if you are under any kind of stress.

B_6 is also important in the body's utilization of fat, which is why a deficiency will produce a rash of skin problems. And it appears that B_6 may play a part in preventing hardening of the arteries; at least Dr. Henry Schroeder, one of the world's leading trace-mineral authorities, has produced this disease state by keeping lab animals on a diet lacking it.

It seems doubtful that sufficient B_6 can be obtained through food alone by anyone under real stress, which certainly defines anyone active in any sport. According to Dr. Schroeder, the processing of milk, meat, the cooking and stewing of foods, result in substantial losses of this vitamin. About half of it goes down the drain when grain is milled, for instance, and processing destroys most of the B_6 in food, although fresh produce generally is high in B_6. A large number of drugs also interfere with the uptake of this water-soluble nutrient.

Meat contains meaty quantities of B_6, for instance, but

only until it's cooked. Since meat is almost never eaten raw, it isn't a good source of B_6, after all.

B_6 is also destroyed by canning and long storage.

Higher than normal amounts of B_{12} or cobalamin are needed by the athlete. "B_{12}," says Ludwig Prokop, "has specific effects on the metabolism of amino acids and the nervous system, especially for athletes performing at high altitudes."

And since levels of B_{12} in the blood decrease with advancing age, the older you are the greater your need for B_{12} supplementation.

B_{12} (technically known as cobalamin) was synthesized in Switzerland in 1948. It is the only known vitamin that has the mineral cobalt as part of its formula and also contains phosphorus and nitrogen. It is necessary for the normal metabolism in the nervous tissue and is involved in protein, fat, and carbohydrate metabolism.

Will your diet give you enough?

Milk and meat are high in B_{12}, but it is unstable (forty to ninety percent, for instance, is destroyed in evaporated milk).

The instability of B_{12} is a problem, but the instability of the receiving body is an even bigger problem. B_{12} is unique among the vitamins in that even the very small quantities needed will not be obtained if the small intestine doesn't absorb them. And B_{12} cannot be absorbed without the presence of gastric juice that contains the "intrinsic factor." Malformation of the colon can prevent this, as can a condition such as diarrhea, sprue, colitis, or a lack of iron. Certain drugs such as antibiotics can disrupt the intestinal environment and prevent absorption.

Despite the propaganda of meat eaters, meat is not the sole source of B_{12}. "Sprouted seeds and grains are exceedingly high in B_{12}," says herb expert Ben Charles Harris. Chlorophyll is one of the finest repositories of the vitamin if you are a vegetarian; so are seaweeds and soybean paste (miso), and in lieu of liver pills to beef up your B_{12} supplies, you could substitute fresh sprout-filled salads every day plus 8–10 ounces of freshly pressed green juice cocktails: celery, parsley, lettuce, comfrey, spinach, etc.

Ralph Bircher says whole grains are a good source of B_{12}, too, despite the widespread fear of B_{12} deficiencies from following strict vegan diets that rule out eggs and milk as well as meat and fish.

Sociologist Rene Dubos speculates that the reason so many vegans thrive on diets apparently low in B_{12} is that bacterial synthesis of the vitamin takes place in the human intestine, much as it does in sheep and other animals. And a healthy intestine probably doesn't need to "psyche up" on meat to start such synthesis.

Vitamin E (Tocopherol)

Tocopherol rhymes with geritol, but there the similarity ends.

"I credit vitamin E (tocopherol) with my endurance to work fourteen hours a day seven days a week," says nutritionist Carleton Fredericks, "I gave it to the Kansas City Athletics when I was a consultant to them. . . ."

"There is good evidence that vitamin E . . . improves stamina," says gerontologist Richard Passwater. "I insist that all my athletes take it."

Vitamin E is the athletes' Grade-A hedge against energy depletion, according to *Meganutrient* author H. L. Newbold. "Some of my patients," says Newbold, "take as much as 4,200 I.U. daily and feel let down as soon as they reduce their dose level."

Numerous experiments have centered around tocopherol's ability to maximize energy output. Studies have demonstrated that high doses of tocopherol considerably improved lung control of oxygen. In 1974, the *Los Angeles Times* reported on experiments conducted by Dr.

Thomas Packard in which lung cells that normally reproduce themselves only 50 times before wearing out reproduced themselves up to 120 times when injected with vitamin E.

And as a plus, E has even demonstrated an ability to improve alertness and learning ability, not so piddling a plus if you're trying to put the whammy on an opponent's more persuasive inner game of tennis.

Probably no vitamin gets straight As like E. But if not administered continuously, it leaves the blood stream in three days. And E needs a supply of A and C plus the sulphur-containing amino acids to do its best work.

Its work includes improving the metabolism of carbohydrates, fats and proteins. The need for oxygen in the body is reduced markedly by vitamin E. It also has an anti-blood-clotting ability. It improves impaired circulation by dilating the blood vessels, promoting a "timed-release" vigor to the body, and often increases physical endurance by more than 50 percent.

Vitamin E, according to the Shute Institute in London, Canada, "may improve muscle power per se, as many studies on athletes, dogs, and horses attest."

E also promotes proper sugar uptake and storage by the muscles, improves blood circulation, and prevents disorders of the blood vessels and heart. "Vitamin E and the B complex are formidable weapons against heart disease," says Carleton Fredericks.

In the opinion of many medical observers, tocopherol does for the body nutritionally what exercise does for it physically: keeps it from wearing out so fast, keeps it looking good a little longer.

You can get "up" with E three ways:

According to the editors of *Health Survival Digest* in a special report on this vitamin,[4] E can be found in these basic forms: man-made natural, succinate-acid salt, and synthetic. Which to use?

"Unless your body has the ability to convert the

synthetic dextro-d-l-tocopherol to the natural dextro-alpha type, synthetic E can not easily enter into any bodily chemical functions. The concentrated and therefore the most effective form of E is the man-made "natural" dextro alpha or d-l-alpha tocopherol." So says Dr. Harold Rosenberg.[5]

He further advises that although many nutritionists suggest taking a mixed capsule because E is found in nature in a mixed state, this form is only beneficial if the capsule contains sufficient d-alpha tocopherol. All this is not quite the contradiction in terms it seems. All vitamin E is the result of considerable processing. But man-made natural is derived from a natural source, that is, soybean, wheat, safflower, corn, and peanuts. Synthetic vitamin E (*dl*-tocopherol) is manufactured through a biochemical process. It is less concentrated, contains less of the more biologically active portions of this vitamin complex, and is considered the less desirable. All vitamin E however, before being packaged and sold, goes through dozens of chemical procedures and "unlike refined foods," says *Health Survival Digest,* "which lose their nutritional values by being overly processed, the therapeutic value of vitamin E depends on how much it has been processed."

Dr. H. L. Newbold, on the other hand, thinks you'd do well to cover all your bets and take both "synthetic" and "natural" forms.

Another nutritionist, W. D. Currier, recommends taking E in the dry powdered form because as a liquid (that includes capsules) it is antagonistic to other supplements you may be taking such as hormone preparations or iron. And since the body does not absorb more than 20–30 percent of what E it does take in and does not store E as it does A, you would do well to dose yourself on the high side.

"When vitamin E is acting as a general antioxidant, it 'sacrifices' itself. Even though vitamin C and some other compounds can recharge E, it definitely can be consumed rapidly and must be replaced in quantities considered excessive in terms of normal vitamins. Ideal intake of vitamin E approaches the ideal intake of C; both are more than just vitamins," says Dr. Passwater.[6]

And if you'd like to super up your C, thereby creating a double upper, remember to couple ascorbic acid and vitamin E in your diet. Because, like vitamin E and EFA, together they strengthen the ability of the tissues to take up oxygen, restore faulty circulation in the blood vessels and small capillaries and help restore normal permeability of the blood vessels.

E is intimately involved in electron transport and other forms of energy utilization and transport. It also is a companion nutrient to vitamin F, an "inseparable relationship" that . . . "holds out the hope that we can increase our energy, nervous health and endurance."

Amen. And what comes after E?

Vitamin F, better known as the essential fatty acids (EFA).

Its role is to form the sex and adrenal hormones, promote valuable intestinal bacteria, and enter into the fat-containing portion of every cell's structure. In an interesting hand-in-hand fashion, these unsaturated fats help your body to use saturated fats.

Fatty acids facilitate the passage of oxygen via the blood stream to all cells, tissues, and organs and are of great importance to respiration and oxygenation of vital organs.

They cooperate in the body with Vitamin D in making calcium available to the tissues and aid in assimilation of organic phosphorus and in proper functioning of the thyroid.

And vitamin F (which is found in rich supply in wheat germ oil) is a partner in good deeds with vitamin E. Foods richest in lecithin are also good sources of vitamin F (egg yolks, soybeans, etc).

According to Dr. A. L. Tappel, of the University of California, in an article on lipids and their oxidation, you can eat linoleic acid by the bucket and not benefit by it without accompanying doses of vitamin E. The problem is easy to avoid if you stick to vegetable oils that have not been hydrogenated because both of these elements occur in any natural oil.

An illustration of how essential these essential fatty acids are?

Numerous studies show that when test animals were forced to use up the supply of EFA that they had stored, a long process since the body holds onto those supplies tenaciously, the animals became seriously ill.

Supermarket salad oils, alas, are no bargain. They are processed to such a point that the lecithin and vitamin E are refined right out of them, and because they are hydrogenated (hydrogen is added to the essential fatty acids), their health-building value is destroyed.

The best source of linoleic acid is safflower oil, which is twice as rich roughly as corn oil, and cottonseed oils, which contain from 35 to 70 percent EFA.

According to Dr. Paul Wren, a Norwegian medical researcher, a tablespoon a day of purified linseed oil can prevent clot-caused heart attacks. (This, however, is not the linseed that is available in paint-supply stores, but the edible linseed that is sometimes known as flaxseed.) The probable reason is that linoleic acid, which linseed has lots of, is rich in a blood platelet anti-adhesiveness agent.

Dr. Newbold recommends 2 tablespoons of safflower oil daily, taken on salad greens or straight from a spoon. Oil that is heated for cooking has lost some of the very qualities you are taking it for.

Vitamin A

Nor can you get to first base before or even along with the rest of the pack if your cup doth not run over (at least by FDA standards) with vitamin A, which is more than just a hedge against infections and night-blindness.

For instance, vitamin A is especially useful in helping

the body to use protein, says the *N.Y. State Journal of Medicine* (January 15, 1964). Although it does not rank as high as some of the "sporting vitamins." Saturating the tissues with A and B stimulates *all* the body secretions, and acts as a "downer," too, since this combination seems to quell nervousness. And whatever A you are taking will go further if it has sufficient companionship from B_2, B_{12} and E.

A tends to come and go even faster than C. According to a Scandinavian researcher, Dr. A. E. Schjoth, "Vitamin A is drained way from body stores faster than other vitamins. Some people lose it just by standing." [7]

Dr. Schjoth found that the slightest of exertions, just ordinary office work, for instance, created significant losses of the vitamin.

Writer Brenda Lewin says, "Researchers have proven that any activity up to four hours from taking A will reduce its absorption." And Richard Passwater adds, "Some people such as professional athletes might require 75,000 to 100,000 USP units of A a day."

You know about liver as a superior source of A, but did you know that natural palm oil and chili peppers are phenomenally rich sources of this vitamin, too? Since A is fairly fragile, the dangers of toxicity are therefore greatly overrated. A is *not* readily absorbed in *any* of its forms, but it is taken up least well in its nonanimal forms, which would include capsules of palmitate, grass, or carotene. Since provitamin A (carotene) is the most readily oxidized and destroyed of all the forms, carrot juice would not be a dependable source of A from day to day. Synthetic forms of vitamin A, based on distilled petroleum by-products, are potentially the most hazardous forms and have been the product used in almost all the dozen known cases of vitamin A poisoning on the books.

And why do many nutritionists warn you that vitamin A taken before bedtime is as ill advised as a cup of coffee?

Because it has stimulating properties. So to get double value out of your daily A, why not take it when you need a little revving up!

A should always be taken with vitamin D because neither is as effective alone. And fortunately, if your input of E is adequate, but your supply of A isn't, the excess E will stimulate the body's uptake of A.

In addition to its well-known role as a night-blindness antidote (a plus if you're a twilight runner or a night-paddle addict), vitamin A is equally important in discouraging respiratory infections and retarding aging, according to Oswald A. Roeks, professor of nutrition at Columbia University.[8]

A deficiency can also result in atrophy of the adrenal glands. In highest-performance conditions, athletes should increase their intake of A to twice the normal dose, according to Dr. Ludwig Prokop. "This has meaning for the mastery of performance because of the central position of the adrenals in the stress system." [9]

Just repeat that every time you have to master another slice of vitamin-A-rich fresh liver, and you'll be A-OK.

Minerals

What about minerals, the electrolytes of your life? Would you go into orthomolecular orbit to improve your game?

To the athlete, the most important ones, those that strongly influence his muscular action and oxygen consumption, are sodium, calcium, phosphorus, magnesium, potassium, and iron.

Mineral metabolism is not simpler than vitamin metabolism, but it is as important, if not more so. It has been estimated that the human body contains 5 pounds of minerals and only one-quarter ounce of vitamins. Minerals must be supplied by your diet, because your body has no other way of producing them. Once supplied, they must be joined by a sufficient amount of ascorbic acid, or else they won't be deposited in your bones where they should be.

Those minerals known as "electrolytes" are especially important to the athlete because they play a key part in preventing cramps and fatigue.

Disabling leg cramps may indeed be the dirty work of low levels of various chemical elements such as sodium chloride and potassium, according to tennis-playing Dr. Robert Leach.

And the minerals you take should be chelated. This is a process by which the minerals are combined in a chemical process with a protein, which is the way minerals occur naturally in the food we eat. It assures that essentially all the minerals will be absorbed, everything else being equal.

"If you take just plain iron or calcium or phosphorus or magnesium, then 80 to 95 percent of that passes out through the intestinal tract," says W. D. Currier. And don't bolt them down on an empty stomach if you want proper absorption.

All the electrolytes, not just sodium, are lost in large amounts when you exercise, resulting eventually in what's known as "sweat debt."

High-potassium rather than high-sodium supplementation are just what sports doctors order nowadays. According to American researchers James Schamaden and W. D. Snively, "High salt intake accelerates sweating, and any initial relief is offset by the deficiency in body reserves (especially of potassium) which it produces shortly thereafter." Actually, say some nutritionists, that not uncommon gotta-have-tossed-salad-or-a-juicy-peach feeling after a game is an expression of depressed potassium levels. (Most fruits and leafy greens are high in potassium.)

The importance of potassium is illustrated by the studies of Professor Bohmer of West Germany, who found that body stores of potassium were lowered by exercise even as the intracellular potassium went up and the extracellular supply went down. A marathoner, he pointed out, may lose 9-12 liters of sweat containing 5-7 mg. of potassium per liter. This is in addition to urinary losses of potassium.

According to Dr. Stanley Schuman, professor of epidemiology at the Medical University of South Carolina, "Without potassium, muscles can't contract, the heart can't beat properly, the nerves can't carry impulses properly. There is absolutely no doubt that bad diets cause potassium deficiency, and this causes illness because when we perspire profusely, the mineral is carried out of the body."

Potassium, like sodium, is a stimulant. Potassium deficiency presents these symptoms: gas, indigestion, low blood sugar, weakened muscles, and degeneration of the heart muscles—which should be enough to scare you off a salted-nut addiction (sodium) into an orange juice habit (potassium).

Just as calcium and magnesium work together, so, too, are sodium and potassium partners in good health. With a marked imbalance in your sodium-potassium levels, there is abnormal response to stimulation on the part of the nerves. "Potassium," as one nutritionist observed, "plays an immense role in muscle motility."

If you care about your ion equilibrium, you might include seaweed in your diet. It's one of the best sources of dietary potassium. Kelp, for instance, is a seaweed containing roughly 11 percent mg. potassium to its 6 percent sodium. Apricots, too, especially dried ones, are superior sources of this mineral. Seaweed is eaten in the Orient as well as in Ireland, Denmark, Norway, Iceland and Scotland.

Among the fruits, those that offer the best balance of potassium to sodium are dried apricots, dried figs, and, among vegetables, beets, raw carrots, celery, Brussels sprouts and snap beans.

Since every natural foodstuff eaten or drunk contains

salt, from a raw pear to a pitcher of beer, replenishment of lost salt in maintaining the body's fluid balance is far less critical than was previously supposed unless you're obese or otherwise out of shape.

Too much sodium interferes with the absorption and utilization of other necessary elements, including protein, and holds up the elimination of uric acid. In the right amount, it can relax the muscles, and in partnership with potassium, keeps your water-retention level on the level.

Real sea salt contains thirty trace minerals, including magnesium, calcium, phosphorus, etc. You can spurn salt altogether if you substitute just kelp, ground cress, mustard sprouts, or something more ambitious like Vegesalt Supersport Salts. (See recipes.)

Runner Bill Gookin, the originator of "Gookinade," an electrolyte replacement drink, says overweight athletes lose three times as much sodium as their Slim Jim counterparts. The sweat of fit runners, he reports, is more dilute, indicating that the well-conditioned body conserves electrolytes more efficiently.

Other researchers in the sodium-supplementation opposition include Dr. Kenneth Cooper of the Aerobics Institute, who believes that it is chiefly magnesium that is most rapidly sweated away with the stress of training and competing. "It is possible," speculates Cooper, "that the cells release potassium easier than magnesium, or magnesium flushes out of the system faster."

"Mild magnesium deficiency may be widespread," Roger Williams reports, "and a disastrous deficiency may not be uncommon among those suffering from heart attacks."

Magnesium has a profound effect on the functioning of your heart. It spares the cells of the heart from damage when oxygen supply is reduced, prevents cholesterol build-up, and tends to keep the calcium-phosphorus balance on an even keel.

Suspect a deficiency if you are bothered by an irregular heart beat, muscle spasms, twitching, tremors, weakness. "If you take vitamins and don't get a lift, or if you get a lift from vitamins that later fades, chances are you need more magnesium," advises Dr. H. C. Newbold.

Magnesium is a major mineral needed for energy. Doctors who treat athletes, report that a magnesium drain is an energy drain, causing fatigue in even the most superbly conditioned athlete. In a test on extremely fatigued patients, Dr. P. E. Formica reported that 87 percent showed dramatic improvement in just four to ten days on magnesium.

If B_1 in big doses has been a bomb, maybe a mineral like magnesium or iron can come to your rescue.

And note that the more protein you eat, the more magnesium you need, say the authors of a 1971 *Prevention* magazine study. If you don't get it, you ultimately run the risk of a calcium and protein deficiency, too. And if you are an ardent eater of enriched bread and polished rice, you ought to be having a side dish of figs, nuts and seeds, apples, or wild rice. The latter whole foods are good magnesium sources, while the enriched products have had 80 percent of their magnesium removed.

"Magnesium," adds the respected Edmond Bordeaux Szekely, author of *The Book of Minerals,* "is a very important ingredient of the green coloring matter in plants (chlorophyll). Magnesium helps in the use of fat in the diet."

How much magnesium should you take to feel good, better, best? According to Dr. Harold Rosenberg, author of the *Doctor's Book of Vitamin Therapy,* 400–800 mg. is good, with older people, large-bodied folks, and the anemic, nervous, and depressed taking the upper limits. If you are large, nervous *and* old, you may even want to shoot for 1,000 mg.

Dr. H. L. Newbold's rx, on the other hand, is to take a

teaspoon of dolomite powder (which also contains calcium in the proper balance) three times a day in a glass of water.

IRON

Iron-deficiency anemia can be even more serious than television commercials would have you believe, especially if you are an athlete. According to Professor W. Halden, in his report to the World Congress for Nutritional Research, anemia may cause degenerative changes in the heart and blood vessels due to insufficient oxygen supply to the tissues by the red blood corpuscles.

Desiccated liver is indisputably the best source of dietary iron and of great importance as a supplement for women who do anything more strenuous than drive to the supermarket. According to Dr. Miguel Layrisse, chief of the Department of Experimental Medicine of the Venezuelan Institute for Scientific Investigation in Caracas, the only iron that is properly assimilated by the body is heme iron, occurring only in products of animal origin.

Heme is the form in which red-blooded animals store more than 80 percent of the iron in their bodies as hemoglobin, the matter that gives blood its color and transports oxygen from the lungs to all the tissues that constantly require it. Liver, nutrition writer Harald Taub points out, "is the richest storehouse of iron in any animal's body because it contains the greatest amount of blood and also because additional reserves are stored in the liver. As a result, when we supplement our diets with dessicated liver, we not only receive approximately ½ mg. of iron with each gram but we receive it in its most absorbable form."

Too much nonheme iron can be dangerous, too. Which makes iron taken in its most natural form all the more valuable since it is balanced with other minerals and naturally contains less iron. Synthetic forms such as ferrous or ferric salt can kill by building up in the system. According to the CPSC,[10] there were 31 deaths and 543 illnesses from iron-overdosing in children over a three-year period from 1969 to 1972. Iron, when it is in an unnatural form like this, tends to be extremely irritating for some users as it passes through the digestive tract.

What does iron, properly taken and properly absorbed, do for you out there on the playing fields?

Iron is used by the bone marrow to manufacture red blood cells. Iron is formed into heme, and the heme is formed into hemoglobin. It is the hemoglobin that in the lungs exchanges carbon dioxide for fresh oxygen, which is then carried to every cell in the body. Moreover, in order to breathe properly, you must have healthy enzymes, in particular the enzyme catalase, which is not formed without sufficient iron.

Sufficient iron means 1 mg. for men and 1.8 mg. for women. Roughly speaking, that is what you use up. Maybe.

If you are a coffee drinker, however, you may be tucking away considerably less iron that you think since caffeine has a tendency to interfere with iron absorption. Also, the EDTA added to canned foods and used in the processing of frozen vegetables and other refined foods prevents the absorption of up to 50 percent of the iron in the food you eat.

Besides operating as the backbone of your breathing apparatus, iron is part of your energy ignition system, too. Enough of it must be available because the cells use oxygen to burn glucose in order to produce energy. Which is why iron deficiency causes oxygen deficiency and produces symptoms such as tiring easily and recovering slowly from exertion.

A daily intake of liver, however, assures you of a full spectrum of B vitamins, a number of other minerals in addition to iron, and a variety of trace minerals, those tremendous trifles, and other unknown nutritional factors. According to Dr. Benjamin Ershoff, liver has been shown to counteract the adverse effects of large doses of toxic drugs, from aspirin to DES.

In powder form, liver can be incorporated into meat broths, gravies, vegetable cocktails, juices, sauces, even dark breads.

George Bernard Shaw, though a vegetarian, took liver, which he called "my medicine." But if as a vegetarian (or a liver hater) you demand your iron in a nonanimal form, here are some sources: organic unsulphured dried apricots, lettuce, parsley, leeks, carrots, cherries (preferably dried), Concord grapes, and avocados.

Science reporter Dorothy V. Harris recommends that women consider oysters, which to her mind are the next best thing to liver as a source of natural iron.

If not oysters, then maybe the budding girl athlete should at least figure some baked beans, dates, or prunes into her meal plans. Girls require twice as much iron as boys once puberty sets in, and the amount of iron stored by the female adult is only 250 mg. compared to 850 mg. for the adult male.

Furthermore, Harris writes, "Recent studies suggest that women who engage in strenuous activity may need iron supplements more than the average woman."

Specifically, she notes:

In a study conducted at Penn State by Emily Haymes (currently at the University of Colorado) and myself, 25% of the women playing in the U.S. National Field Hockey Tournament were deficient in iron. We also found that 32% of the moderately active women in the State College, Pennsylvania, area were iron-deficient, while only 8% of the sedentary women tested were deficient. . . ." [11]

Don't let iron deficiency anemia leave you breathless.

CALCIUM

Calcium is the "take heart" mineral. It improves the general muscular activity of the heart, often lowers levels of cholesterol and other damaging fats, puts a brake on high blood pressure, and prevents other heart abnormalities.

It is also among the four "most missing nutrients" cited in the Department of Agriculture's surveys of the American diet. In contrast to iron, you cannot "O.D." on calcium, says Dr. Harold Rosenberg.[12] But what you take is not necessarily what you get. "The average person tends not to absorb calcium very well ..." says biochemist Richard Pardee, "Perhaps ... 10% to 20% of that found in the foods eaten."

On a high-protein diet, advises Dr. H. L. Newbold, approximately 15 percent of the calcium taken by mouth is absorbed. Furthermore, strenuous exercise creates a greater need for extra calcium.

A number of things impair your absorption of calcium. A high-fat diet will do it, since those fats form insoluble calcium soaps in the intestinal tract, causing the calcium to pass through unabsorbed. So do antacids and bicarbonate of soda. The calcium in certain vegetables may not be properly released because of the oxalates found naturally in rhubarb, cauliflower, spinach, and a similar situation exists with grains that contain phytates that block assimilation.

Dr. Newbold continues:

Low-protein diets (which is another way of designating the rich-in-refined-carbohydrates diet so common in our society) assure an absorption of only 5%, and refined sugars act to block the absorption of calcium in much the same way. An insufficiency of hydrochloric acid in the gut is another limiting factor in the absorption of calcium (and iron).

Calcium comes from some uncommon sources. There is calcium in stone, bone, wheat, and even sugar before they are refined. Mexican peasants get calcium from limestone. It migrates into their cornmeal when the grain is pounded into flour. Eskimos get calcium from the fish bones they eat along with the flesh.

Another way of getting and absorbing more calcium may be to adopt vegetarianism. At least the *American Journal of Clinical Nutrition* has reported that vegetarians, even those who do not drink milk, have bones of greater density than those of meat eaters. Salad greens may be a better calcium source than pasteurized milk, after all.

According to biochemist Richard Pardee the best form of calcium to take is calcium phosphate, because "the phosphate has a hydrogen bond, and the principal calcium of the body is calcium hydrogen phosphate." Pardee advises calcium lactate as the second-best-absorbed type.

A third recommended source of calcium is bonemeal, which has an excellant calcium-phosphorus ratio. The ideal is something like 2½ to 1½ calcium to one of phosphorus.

One way to spoon feed yourself calcium and magnesium, another much-needed mineral, is to take 3 teaspoons of dolomite daily, thereby providing yourself with 1,180 mg. of calcium and 700 mg. of magnesium simultaneously.

Other vitamins and minerals, amino acids, or related trace elements that provide a "natural hormonal high" for some of the weekend athletes among us include:

Aspartic acid, of which Dr. Roger Williams says,

One means of determining stamina is to force an animal to swim until exhausted ... and note the swimming time. It is by this means that it has been found recently that the amino acid aspartic acid is possibly of greater nutritional importance than had been previously suspected. Administering salts of this acid to rats is reported to double the length of time they can swim before exhaustion. Corroboration of this increase in stamina has been reported in the case of . . . athletes . . . also. Aspartic acid, if you'd like to go on a binge, is readily available in foods such as almonds, apricots, lemons and watercress.

And Dr. H. L. Newbold suggests another amino acid to try if you want to pull yourself up by your jockstraps: glutamine, which constitutes the bulk of nourishment for your nervous system (along with glucose).

If you've had a tough time getting off the not-so-safe uppers and downers, a "healthy high" might come your way by way of glutamine (not to be confused with glutamic acid, which is a supplement of a different order). It is definitely stimulating. Taken a capsule or two at a time, says Dr. H. L. Newbold, "it can be overstimulating." It is uplifting and seems completely safe.

If you'd like to try glutamine—there are no reported cases of unfavorable side effects—the recommended dose is one 200 mg. capsule three times daily. Take it with meals if you find it too stimulating. Double your dosage if you're getting good results.

And then there is an adjunct to any diet that really does it. A kind of diet "rider" that packs a lot of punch for some weekend athletes. Dr. Hans Kugler, a tennist and equestrian, calls it the nucleic acid cure.

Every three to four months I take about 1,200 to 2,000 mg. of a nucleic acid preparation three to four times per week. After the three weeks I take only 200 mg. three to four times per week. Whenever I take large quantities of nucleic acids I drink a lot of liquids to prevent any effects from the metabolites of nucleic acids.

If you are fortunate enough to have found a heads-up holistic physician, it could be just such a cure that will help you realize your performance.

Downers

And are vitamins, minerals, and herbs also useful as downers? You bet your sweet sleep life they are. The herb zendo is a natural appetite depressant; B_6 and calcium are tranquilizers; the amino acid tryptophan is practically a sleeping pill, and exercise itself is not only an energizing aid but a sleep inducer as well. Who among us has not discovered the joy of sleeping after a two-mile run and a glass of warm milk?

According to William G. DeLameter, Ph. D., "Lecithin rather than sleeping pills should be taken by the individual whose nerves are shot."

Nodding assent on the nodding-off issue is osteopath Dr. Albert C. Pietsch, "Lecithin enables the brain to work with greater intensity and for longer hours, and better normal sleep is the result."

After all, turning yourself off is just as important as turning yourself on. If you aren't relaxed and well rested, you can't play at the peak of your powers. One reason may be that important B vitamins are synthesized only during deep (S-type) sleep.

One food-based sleep-tight trick comes from the American Federation for Clinical Research, which points out that the amino acids in the blood stream dramatically affect ability to sleep. If they're depleted, sleep is difficult. Behavior is also affected. The secret to getting the essential amino acids? Ingest fresh protein (eggs, milk, natural cheese, raw nuts, whole grains, beans, fish, poultry and meat, etc.).

Other experts remind the semiserious athlete that upsetting the amino acid equilibrium in the blood by changing your food intake too radically can also affect the way you sleep and even alter your brain functions. In other words, improper protein input can derange your sleep appestat as well as your hunger appestat.

Research shows that high-stress foods, too, can keep you unpleasantly hyped up. So deemphasize vittles like fried chicken, French fries, even ice cream and dried fruit in large amounts, all of which elevate blood fat levels, blood pressure, and resting pulse rates.

Another sleeper is the B vitamin inositol, "a moderate-to-mild tranquilizer–sedative," says Dr. Robert C. Atkins; and Dr. Carl Pfeiffer uses it in 2,000-mg. doses to lower blood pressure. This amount at bedtime should send you off to the land of nod, while a lesser amount (650 mg.) makes an effective and 100 percent-safe daytime sedative.

In the appetite "downers" department, ketones are another drugless downer. The more you've got circulating, the less hungry you feel. You can get your ketones and energy up—while getting your hunger levels down by fasting or by a high-protein, very low carbohydrate diet of the type such as Dr. Robert C. Atkins advocates in his many books.

But exercise may be all you need to unwind. According to Herbert P. DeVries, Ph. D., California exercise physiologist, volleyball is a better downer than valium, especially for aging athletes. DeVries has demonstrated that simply taking a 15-minute walk produces more muscular relaxation than any kind of tranquilizer.

Cardiologist Dr. Paul White is also a believer in the superiority of exercise in the relaxacisor department. "The leg muscles," he says, "are an important and unappreciated accessory pumping mechanism to assist our hearts physically. Healthy fatigue of the great muscle is the best antidote known to man for nervous stress. . . ."

Numerous herbs promote sleep, and stress can be a tempest in a teapot if your teapot is full of soothing herbs.

Damiana is described as a good relaxant and nervine by herbalists. *Peppermint,* too, is a downer. And anybody who's read *Peter Rabbit* knows chamomile's reputation as a garden-patch barbiturate.

Take a soporific tea and see for yourself. Here's one such to mix after your match.

> 1 dry ounce dried peppermint leaves (a digestive)
> 1 tablespoon rosemary leaves (a tranquilizer)
> 1 tablespoon sage leaves (a soporific)

Mix and store in tightly closed jar. Use one tablespoon of the mixture to a cup of boiling water. Let steep for one minute, strain, sweeten with honey, and sip. Fortify with milk if you're bed bound.

Vitamin Needs

How can you determine the vitamin needs for your sporting life? One way is to weigh what you're eating. Whatever that is will be eating up a good part of your vitamin rations as well. Drugs of any kind (and that includes caffeine, nicotine, alcohol and chemical sugar substitutes) destroy large amounts of the entire B complex. Oddities like raw shellfish destroy the B_1 and B_{12} in your system, and your supply of C is routinely wiped out by everything from a mild cold to a heated battle over who won the last point. There are numerous culprits that C gets used up by and that upset the body's acid-alkaline balance: shocks, keen disappointments, intense emotional upsets, excessive fears, overworking, overtraining and underresting, according to Linda Clark.

The world's foremost authority on stress, Dr. Hans Selye, warns that ascorbic acid supplies in the adrenal glands can be destroyed in seconds.

One outburt of anger, according to Dr. Fred Klenner, [13]

can burn up as much as 3,000 mg. of vitamin C. This puts you considerably in the red if all you've been taking is the government's recommended daily allotment of 45 mg.

All of the fat-soluble vitamins (A, K, E, D) are destroyed by mineral oil, which you may find in your ice cream, along with other unidentified chemicals. Vitamin E is destroyed by the sort of bleaching agents routinely used in white bread and similar processed foods. All the sulfa drugs destroy vitamin K. Nitrites and nitrates in ham, hot dogs and luncheon meats, and vegetables grown with nitrate-rich fetilizers destroy numerous vitamins. If you're a swimmer, a lot of your vitamin E is being destroyed by the chlorine you are inadvertently swallowing and absorbing through your skin.

Then there is that nonspecific: stress.

Russian research has shown that because of stress, "Athletes require additional 'B' and 'C,' at least twice that of the non-athlete. Some coaches and researchers suggest 5 to 10 times more ... and all of them seem to agree that vitamin E, wheat germ oil, and wheat germ should be added to the athlete's diet." [14]

Sugar destroys the amino acid, glutamic acid, and drugs used commonly in treating high blood pressure and Wilson's Syndrome wipe out B_6. Other drugs such as anticonvulsants and oral contraceptives also burn up B_6 and folic acid. Epilepsy drugs create a vitamin D shortage; aspirin, antacids, even activated charcoal, are vitamin depleters.

And there is currently some fear that sorbitol, the artificial sweetener widely used in gums, candies, and dietetic foods, may change the absorption of various drugs you may be taking.

Antibiotics destroy vitamin B in the intestinal tract, and processing procedures like pasteurization destroy the B complex plus minerals.

Injuries and stress take their toll, creating deficiencies,

and even coffee drinking gets minuses here. Lavish amounts of it not only deplete lavish amounts of B and C, but coffee also plays havoc with your body's absorption of dietary iron.

Moral? In the case of vitamins, you should give yourself a generous depletion allowance. What you take is never what you get.

Isn't good food the best source of vitamins? It's doubtful.

From soil to consumption, according to researcher-writers Cheraskin and Ringsdorf, as much as 90 percent of food's value may be lost. Year by year the vitamin content of our food supply keeps declining. From 1944 to 1958, there was a uniform decline in the vitamins available in our food. For vitamin C, 23 percent decline; there was 22 percent less vitamin A available, and 16 percent less B_1.[15] Certainly conditions have worsened rather than improved over the last twenty years, with refined foods making up a greater and greater portion of the American diet.

Important trace elements are lost, too.

"When you refine an honest carbohydrate like wheat, you are removing not only the bran, but 50 to 80 percent of the trace elements which are very important for health," says Dr. Benjamin H. Ershoff.[16] He adds, "I disagree with the FDA. . . . they are 100 percent wrong when they say if you eat a balanced diet you don't need supplements."

Synthetic vitamins are in reality drugs, and they can, in the opinion of many naturopathically oriented doctors, cause some of the same undesirable side effects that drugs do.

Synthetic vitamins have their usefulness, of course. For the food-allergic person they minimize exposure, and provide an alternative to corn, salt, starches, and other allergy-provoking materials commonly used in binding tablets, as well as to the main-ingredient offenders such as brewers yeast, sugar, soy flour, etc.

Some synthetics seem to offer nearly the same benefits of the natural ones or in some cases offer a different but equally valuable benefit. For instance, Dr. Linus Pauling puts his money behind plain ascorbic acid as opposed to naturally derived vitamin C. And Dr. Newbold is one of the many physicians who feel that both synthetic (succinate) and natural (acetate) forms of vitamin E are of equal value.

According to Samuel Syers, on the other hand, vitamin E is an apt example of superiority of the natural over the synthetic. Although the two forms appear identical, polarized light affects them differently. And animal studies show that natural d-alpha tocopherol is 20–36 percent more active than the synthetic dl-tocopherol.

There are a number of other negative factors to consider. Vitamins may contain salt, sugar, artificial colors, allergy-provoking fillers, mineral oil, and bisulfite.

You pays your money and takes your choice.

Exercise

"We must exercise to preserve our health," says Dr. Jesse Steinfeld former surgeon general of the U.S. Public Health Service. "We will sleep better, eat better, digest our food better. . . ."

"If you work out regularly, you'll change jouncy fat to lean muscle—even without changing your diet," says Dr. C. Harmon Brown, medical director of the Student Health Services at California State University. A study of 350 obese subjects revealed that the "onset of obesity was related to inactivity in nearly 70% of the cases; in only 3.2% of the cases was increased food intake related to weight gain." [17]

A nonexerciser never uses more than two-thirds the lung expansion available to him. The heart itself shrinks, its beats become less regular, protein within the muscle cells decreases, utilization of oxygen becomes wasteful and inefficient. You, on the other hand, since you've chosen to bike, hike, hit, kick, or sock something around a chosen course, are in for the following benefits: a slower heart rate, more oxygen available, more fully developed heart-muscle fibers, and, depending on the extent of your training, a larger, heavier heart, greater lung capacity, and an improved ability to recover from any kind of exertion.

Exercise may also improve your resistance to disease, while it increases your sense of general well-being. The oxygen-thin air of high altitudes builds better hearts and stronger arteries. Witness the superior health of the Peruvian Indians. And, says Dr. Raul Gamboa, who is presently conducting a study of these peoples, "Exercise is exactly the same as being at high altitudes."

Exercise is sometimes a life saver. Indeed, many physiologists and nutritionists feel that if you had to choose, you'd be better off with a delinquent diet and a superior exercise program. In a series of Japanese tests with lab animals at the Labor Science Research Institute, the incidence of cancerous livers was lowest in the high-exercise group (23.5) and highest in the low-exercise group.[18]

Exercise also improves self-confidence, according to studies by Purdue University's A. H. Ismail. That isn't surprising when you consider that improved circulation means improved brain function. While lack of exercise allows the blood cholesterol levels to shoot up, sufficient activity burns up excess cholesterol in the body. This means the more active you are, the less you have to fear from high-cholesterol foods, which are quite often the ones that supply optimum nutrition.

But you don't get something for nothing. Haphazard, slapdash nutritional practices can considerably narrow the full extent of such benefits, just as supernutrition can maximize such dividends.

When you are well exercised, your body can actually

double the amount of glycogen it stores in the muscles. In addition, regular exercise allows your bones to become stronger, denser, and more capable of retaining calcium.

But exercise is virtually useless, according to Nathan Pritkin, unless practiced in conjunction with a low-fat diet, which is practically a no-fat diet, as practiced by his Longevity Research Center.

Why? Because says Pritikin, who is a ten-mile-a-morning runner, fat entering the blood stream after a meal lowers the oxygen-carrying capacity of the blood, dulls the mind and senses and causes fatigue.

The reverse is also true. Exercise enhances and maximizes the effect of nutritional supplements such as wheat-germ oil and ascorbic acid in the body.

Moreover, according to reporter Dorothy V. Harris, in December 1977 *WomenSports Magazine,* it appears that "the bone marrow which manufactures blood, actually becomes redder under the influence of exercise. This would seem to indicate an increased blood-forming capacity."

So, don't just sit there.

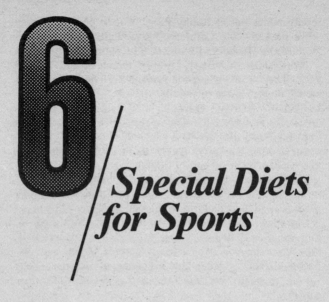

6 / Special Diets for Sports

"Loading" is megadosing with one particular type or class of food for the purpose of raising your performance potential. The special diets discussed here work some of the time for some of the athletes who food trip with them, but none of them work for everybody all of the time. Here are some of the why's and why not's, and if you'd like to try them, the what's what of the most celebrated loading diets.

Protein Loading

Of all the diets that athletes have adopted traditionally, the leader is protein loading.

The Greek Olympians tried to boost their performances by eating protein-rich cheese. And protein in several forms was the food fuse used in recent times to get an Olympic performance out of Bobby Riggs. But its popularity may have peaked. "Most athletes," says Walter Gregg, chairman of the Health and Physical Education Department at Northwestern University, "are off the steak and vitamin kick. They're off it because doctors are convincing them that it doesn't work very well."

Certainly extreme examples of the ultra-high protein-loading diet, such as Bernarr McFadden's milk saturation diet, have had their heyday.

McFadden, author of *The Miracle of Milk,* advocated guzzling 6 quarts of milk a day, thereby contributing 200 extra grams of protein to the diet.

Such eating plans have been succeeded by less extreme high-protein regimens, but for Hollywood nutritionist Rheo Blair, best known as the Svengali behind Bobby Riggs's rejuvenation, protein does have miraculous powers.

It can produce, says Blair, "A more dependable energy level, great complexion, shining hair, and bright clear eyes. . . ."

Predigested proteins, high-protein meals, and concentrated supplements rich in protein such as liver powder and wheat germ oil were a few of the nutriments that made a superman out of Bobby Riggs in only seven weeks. It was augmented by blood circulation stimulation and light exercise.

Such a diet enabled Riggs to beat the lace pants off Margaret Court. "I had the feeling that I could run right through a wall if I wanted to," said Riggs.

Cell regeneration through proteins and amino acids is Blair's basic objective, and Riggs was but one among thousands that the nutritionist has put through the proteinaceous paces.

Many of his ideas are at variance with those of conventional nutritionists. He has little use for vegetable protein or for vegetables or fruits themselves. He omits them because they "take up too much room in the digestive system." Blair himself hasn't eaten bread, vegetables, or fruits for years. Meat, milk, and eggs are the backbone of his feeding program, and he believes that enough protein must be used to not only take care of present needs but to make up for past deficiencies.

Whether you are loading proteins, leaving them out (in favor of carbohydrates), or temporarily ignoring them (as in the "Reversal" or "Live Longer Now" diet), proteins pose some complicated dietary questions.

How much is enough? How much is too much? Do you or don't you need more to perform better?

Recent bulletins from the USDA set the body's minimum protein requirements at 30 to 40 grams each day, considerably lower than a decade ago. Many experts disagree.

According to Richard Pardee, "Personal study and observation show me that 100 to 140 grams of protein daily is not out of line for an active adult." [1]

A study by V. E. Jordon, assistant professor at the University of Maine, points out that new research indicates the body's tissue proteins are not replaced as rapidly as had previously been thought, and physical and emotional stresses tend to limit tissue absorption of protein.

Another recent study indicates that muscle and connective tissue alone require 70 grams of protein for optimum nitrogen utilization, and additional nitrogen is needed for the synthesis of RNA for proper cell function.

Many researchers are in agreement that an additional 20 to 30 grams over the 70 needed for muscle function is a safe bet.

Also on the pro side of the protein question is the noted Dr. Hans J. Kugler:

The best way to assure the right supply of the correct proteins is to eat more than one type of protein at a time. . . . To get enough proteins, you should try to eat at least 20 gms. more per day then recommended.

If you eat too much protein, your body can store a small quantity and will convert excess proteins into sugar . . . .

Dr. Kugler further suggests that "if you take protein preparations, make sure that these preparations contain the essential amino acids and in the right percentages. . . ."

On the con side of the protein question, reporter Peggy Eastman, writing in *Harper's Bazaar,* [2] talks about what she calls the "Protein Myth." "Americans . . . often exceed the RDA set by the National Academy of Science's Food and Nutrition Board. If protein is good for us . . . is more of a good thing better? The answer is 'no' according to a growing body of scientific evidence."

In agreement are two of the world's leading authorities on protein and calcium: Mark Hegstead of Harvard University and Doris Calloway of the University of California at Berkeley. One of the things that's wrong with protein foods in excess, they say, is that they are rich in the three acid-forming minerals sulphur, chlorine, and phosphorus, and too much acid in the body paves the way for illness.

"Less protein," says Dr. Roy L. Walford, working at the University of California at Los Angeles on a grant from the National Institute on Aging, "is actually beneficial. When a low-protein diet is fed to rats, they live 15 to 40 percent longer." And nutritionist Dr. Jean Mayer adds that the exceedingly athletic long-living Hunzas of Pakistan are fueled by a low-protein (35 grams) diet derived mainly from vegetable sources.

Protein loading (which may be defined as an intake of say 142 grams as opposed to a moderate or "normal" daily input of 56) is the level at which osteoporosis developed in men, in tests conducted by Helen M. Linkswiler at the

University of Wisconsin's Department of Nutritional Sciences.[3]

Also, protein loading usually means extra fat intake, which is dangerous because it can create a deficiency of B_6 and magnesium if these nutrients aren't bumped up, too.

If you do decide to dose with protein, don't do it before your doubles match. According to Dr. David Vaughn, chief of the Protein Nutrition Laboratory at the Nutrition Institute, Agriculture Research Service, high levels of protein can be especially dangerous ingested before strenuous exercise. An increased protein intake calls for more water to take care of the increased load of urea coming through the kidneys, and this can put a strain on anybody's kidneys, especially those of the older athlete.

Finally, two more gut issues: Don't overload. The body can only digest 25 grams of protein every three to five hours.

Second, remember that protein needs large amounts of hydrochloric acid to be digested, too, and if you are over forty, you may be HCL-short.

Whether or not you are short of digestive juices or are an older athlete, it is still a good idea to supplement your meals with extra HCL if you are taking in higher levels of protein than 30–40 gm. And whatever you do, let the protein part of your meal precede the salad and the rest. This order allows your stomach to produce the gastric juice necessary to digest the protein that otherwise might remain largely undigested.

But suppose you are a tennis player with a tendency toward gout? Many proteins—sardines, liver, kidney, etc.—have a high-purine content, and according to Dr. Charles H. Barrows, Jr., of the National Institute on Aging, these foods are on the not-recommended list.

On the other hand, inadequate protein intake can be dangerous and have damaging effects on your performance. Anemia may develop due to improper iron absorption, since the oxygen-carrying pigment of the blood is largely made up of protein. There is the possibility too, of developing bone-marrow maladies because protein is necessary in the preformation of bone marrow.

Inadequate protein intake over a long enough period of time can also result in chronic digestive troubles. It also can lead to impaired absorption of vitamin A, which in turn will lower your resistance to infection and your energy.

But if you're eating a diet of natural foods, says Dr. Paavo Airola, it's almost impossible not to get enough protein.

Assuming that you could afford it, protein loading with steak would be a particularly bad idea. Meat travels through the system at a snail's pace and may take up to four hours to get around to your intestinal tract. If it's a pregame meal, the sugars in steak protein are so slowly converted to energy they won't catch up to you until after all the cheering has stopped, anyhow.

Too much protein is not only wasteful but harmful, too. According to Ralph A. Nelson, assistant professor of nutrition at the Medical School of the Mayo Clinic, high-protein intake increases enzymatic activity and the production of urea and albumin, which has the effect of "idling our metabolic engine at a faster rate." A possible reason why women live longer than men, he adds, is that they consume less protein than men.

Reinforcing Dr. Nelson's concerned warnings are researchers at the University of Wisconsin, whose study of subjects on a high-protein diet have demonstrated that if your daily protein intake is very high (90 grams, they mean), you are in for a very substantial loss of calcium, which leaves the body by way of the urinary tract due to acid-ash biochemical interaction of the protein. This puts your body into negative calcium balance and paves the way for osteoporosis, according to Dr. Helen M. Linkswiler.

But doesn't active muscle turnover mean your protein requirement is higher? Most of the evidence concludes it does not.

Despite the link between "steaks and sports," the active athletic body requires little more protein than the inactive unathletic body. The protein requirements of an adult for maintenance of existing tissue is low, about 20 grams, and only slightly more is needed by the athlete. If it is unavailable, little harm is done since the body can live for what Ralph Bircher, director of Switzerland's famed Bircher-Benner Clinic in Zurich, calls "an astonishing long time on its own substance without the slightest harm to organs or muscles."

Consider the harm that comes to the body from protein loading and overloading:

1. Excess protein stresses the kidneys with large amounts of decomposition products that must be quickly eliminated. Postgame studies of players on protein-loading diets show considerable incidence of kidney damage and occasional kidney failure, plus elevated blood pressure levels.
2. Extra protein is indeed stimulating to some people, but it is a temporary lift like that of sugar.
3. Women are in danger of damaging their ovaries and even run the risk of masculinization from a high-protein training diet.

It all adds up to the fact that protein loading may be an idea whose time has come and gone.

High-Carbohydrate Diets and Carbohydrate Loading

Less than 20 percent of our caloric intake these days comes from good old filling carbohydrates.

Dr. Seymour L. Halpren [4] thinks even the unathletic

individual's diet should have more than twice the car-bohydrate content it does; that would mean 50 percent for those who are sitting it out, and 60 percent for you and me, who are out there getting a piece of the action.

Carbohydrate-high diets and carbohydrate loading bring up the question of the conditioned or "acclimatized" versus the unconditioned athlete. A case in point: Mar-athon runners use .9 calorie per kilogram of body weight, while aspiring athletes like you and me doing the same thing use about 1. calorie. Running a marathon will set you back about 2,280 calories if you weigh 60 kilograms.

It is a slight edge, but a carbohydrate-rich diet will allow you to produce a bit more energy for every liter of oxygen: 4.92 for carbohydrate-rich diets, versus 4.86 after mixed diets and 4.8 after fat-rich diets. Which may be why pasta, dried prunes, and mashed potatoes suddenly eclipsed charcoal-broiled steaks and milk shakes at the Olympic Village in Montreal in 1976.

Whether a high-carbohydrate diet prior to your event is appropriate depends on a number of factors.

In *Nutrition for Maximal Sports Performance* Bergstrom and Hultman [5] tell us that "at low intensities of work, energy is mainly derived from lipids. The fraction of carbohydrate used as an energy source increases with increasing work load, with the result that at 85 percent to 90 percent of maximum inspiratory oxygen-volume capac-ity, all energy is derived from carbohydrates."

The authors proceed to recommend this: "While the athlete is in training, he should take a diet which has adequate caloric content (3,000 to 5,000) and is relatively rich in protein."

Dr. David G. Guy, a noted nutritional researcher quoted in *Nutrition for Athletes,* questions the heavy in-clusion of polysaccharides, disaccharides, and monosac-charides (carbohydrates all) in the diet.

It appears from the scientific literature that the more the muscle is worked, the higher the demand for carbohydrate. The diet (carbohydrate-loading) consists of nearly 70% of the calories coming from carbohydrates. Swedish workers have shown that it is possible to increase the fuel level of carbohydrate in the muscle; however this requires very complex dietary manipulation.

You could do some of this starchy stocking up if you live by bread alone for a while, gaining energy and not even winding up with a pumpernickel belly.

In a study conducted by Dr. Olaf Mickelsen of Michigan State University, a group of slightly overweight young men lost an average of 12.7 pounds each over an eight-week period. While eating twelve slices of bread each day. In another study conducted by Dr. Mickelsen, twelve young men obtained from 90 percent to 95 percent of their protein needs from white enriched bread, although the report suggests that whole-wheat bread may "provide more micronutrients and definitely provides more fiber than white bread." [6]

In a nutshell, carbohydrate loading is a technique credited to Per-Olaf Astrand that is used largely by endurance athletes facing a long race or a strenuous event of some duration. To use a runner as an example:

The runner takes his run of say one and a half hours. Over the following three days, he limits his diet to protein foods such as fish, cheese, eggs, and meat and avoids carbohydrates. The next three days, a normal diet is followed but with the addition of as much carbohydrate as the athlete can stand. On the day of the race, the runner has a light meal. The purpose of all this is to deplete the leg muscles of glycogen supplies during the first two stages, allowing the athlete to then "load," binding an enormous amount of carbohydrate to the muscle and promoting markedly increased endurance.

Does it work?

Experiments in Sweden have shown that work capacity could be increased anywhere from 100 to 300 percent and that running time in an 18-mile race could be improved by as much as fifteen minutes. If a loaf of bread can give you an edge like that, it is a very impressive technique indeed.

Likewise, Paul Slovic's studies of fifty loaders at a Trails End Marathon in 1975 showed an average improvement of eight and a half minutes, which translates into twenty seconds or 100 yards per mile.

It also appears that carbohydrates have in their favor an element of efficiency not offered by the other food groups. They are 10 percent more efficient in utilizing the body's oxygen than either fats or proteins are.

As simple and safe as it sounds, there are those who think that stimulating yourself with all that starch to improve performance is a lousy idea.

"Carbohydrate loading is a terrible idea," says the father of the reversal diet, also known as the low-cholesterol, low-fat diet, the "Live Longer Now Diet," and the Complex-Carbohydrate Diet. Says Nathan Pritikin, "Carbohydrate loading is actually fat-loading. The heavy protein is actually heavy fat, and you'll kill yourself in the high-protein period. It's terribly unhealthy. A normal, high-carbohydrate diet means you are storing glycogen in your muscles and liver and you're loaded all the time."[7]

Concurring is runner-M.D. George Sheehan, a heart specialist and no slouch as a runner, who points out that clogged kidneys ending in renal shutdown have also resulted from this kind of loading. "Most likely set in motion by the first three days of low-carbohydrate intake and continued training rather than the three-day binge of carbohydrates that follows. . . ." he speculates.

Additional dangers are in store for the allergic and/or hypoglycemic runner; it is estimated that there are fifty million hypoglycemics in this country. Sheehan, also a low blood sugar victim, points out, "The high rate of blood-sugar expenditure during exercise quickly exhausts an already inadequate reserve of liver glycogen and brings on hypoglycemic stress." So this superupper can be a super-stresser for some. Dr. Sheehan's preventive Rx is to take 2-4 grams of pure fructose hourly between meals to help avoid the mental and emotional depression that occurs during the low-carbohydrate phase. Fructose is thought to help in equalizing the fuel supply because of its slow rate of absorption. Unfortunately, fructose has its minuses, too, as discussed under sugar in the "Junk Food" chapter.

Dr. H. L. Newbold also warns that the carbohydrate loader is skating on thin ice, that significant levels of carbohydrate make the blood-sugar levels erratic all day.

While viewing with a jaundiced eye those protein-packing diets, Dr. Ralph Bircher maintains that a carbohydrate-rich diet and an optimal supply of vitamins, minerals, and trace elements provide alertness, protection from the cold, fuel for action, and various stresses for the ice-hockey pro. And what's a boon to a puck pusher is probably pretty good medicine for a road runner or a rower, too.

Carbohydrates make up most of the world food supply. They are contained in easily grown plants, and 365 grams of carbohydrate provide enough energy to fuel the bodily functions for about thirteen hours.

Carbohydrates also serve special purposes in the vital organs. In the liver, they are oxidized as fuel, while the central nervous system depends on a steady supply of carbohydrates for proper functioning. "Irreversible brain damage may occur as a result of insufficient carbohydrate being supplied to the brain," warn the authors of *Nutrition and the Athlete.*

But carbohydrates are *bad* brain foods in the opinion of Dr. Benjamin Feingold, who reports that studies made on brain biochemistry now appearing in the scientific literature indicate it is this food group, not only sugar but carbohydrates in general, that influences the biochemistry of the brain, and not for the better, either. Said Feingold to a *Let's Live* reporter, [8] "New works such as those coming out of M.I.T. convince me that sugar and *all* carbohydrates may be very serious trouble-causing factors. . . ."

But the observable fact remains that a potato provides more go power than a peanut. Physical work of a given intensity can be continued for an average of four hours without undo stress when an athlete has prepped with potatoes and other carbohydrates rather than fats and proteins. Four times greater energy is yielded.

Not, of course, that either method works wonders for everyone. According to cyclist and editor of *Bike World* George Beinhorn, "On the two unhappy cases I overdid it, eating too much carbohydrate food, my heartbeat and breathing rates increased, making sleep shallow and unrestful and sapping the energy I would have used to race."

But Swedish physiologist Bengt Saltin insists that pre-race diets, rich during the last three days in spaghetti, pie, potatoes, and the like and carbohydrate-poor the week before a race, work wonders.

Even a three-day, carbohydrate-rich diet often results in an improvement in endurance of 50 percent, says Per-Olaf Astrand, the technique's originator.

And since many participants find that the week of no carbohydrates is stressful and tiring, the answer is yes, it is possible to skip this phase, although results will not be as dramatic. You can try just the loading phase of the diet, carried out for three days before the contest you are psyching for. In this case, the guidelines are: (1) Make sure your last four to six meals are carbohydrate heavy, (2) begin the diet after a lengthy training session, and (3) do very little training during the dietary period.

Partial loaders, observes Paul Slovic, rarely have the difficulties cited by loaders who go all the way.

Then there is a complex carbohydrate diet that really doesn't get into loading at all—the low-fat, low-cholesterol diet? Will it give you the run for your money you're after?

Although many experts in sports nutrition point to evidence that energy emanates largely from a healthy intake of either fats or carbohydrates, the "Reversal Diet" has many partisans. Given by nutritional scientist Nathan Pritikin at his Longevity Research Institute, it is a drastic low-fat diet eliminating all dairy products, most meats, and all fatty fishes. When combined with a controlled exercise routine, it supposedly produces astounding changes within a few weeks, increasing blood flow and raising the blood's rate of oxygen consumption.

It is called the "Reversal Diet" because it "reverses" the condition of high-cholesterol, high-blood fats. When they're low enough in the blood stream, the arteries begin to open again.

And Pritikin emphasizes the very foods that Blair's high-protein diet eliminates: vegetables, fruits, and grains. Yet Pritikin is just as firmly convinced as Blair that "restoring the circulation" or improving it is the name of the game. Although the greatest successes so far have been with heart patients anxious to "reverse" their conditions through diet and exercise, on a Pritikin-supervised, low-cholesterol, low-fat diet Eula Weaver came back from her deathbed to win four medals as a runner at the Senior Olympics at the age of eighty-eight.

It is being adopted by cyclists, runners, and other athletes, too, in the hopes of getting a little closer to that elusive but achievable "superself."

Vegetarianism

You don't have to be a pig sticker to be a pigskin kicker anymore.

If you would prefer not to live and perform by pork chop alone, you're in good company. The North American Vegetarian Society estimates that one out of every twenty Americans is on some sort of nonflesh-foods diet these days. Among them, for instance, is Bill Walton, and if he can make it without Big Macs, who are you to scorn a plant-centered diet?

Being on the lam from lamb is not a new idea. There are a lot of precedents for such a life style, and a lot of alternatives to ball park redhots and the thick steaks that coaches and the not-so-well-informed common man are still so uncommonly fond of.

So what's so wrong with good red meat, anyway? According to Dr. Benjamin Frank, "Meats have the most detrimental effect (on performance), for they are low in nucleic acid and high in sluggishly metabolized cholesterol and fats.... In light sports, vegetarianism has a special value for athletes."

"A vegetarian," says the National Academy of Sciences, "can be well nourished if he eats a variety of plant foods and gives attention to critical nutrients." Meat is a known stimulant containing large quantities of uric acid (dioxypurine), which yields more energy initially but tends to taper off after a relatively short time. So don't turn to meat to get a buzz on. It has the same short-term disadvantages of sugar, drugs, caffeine, Coca Cola, and foods concocted therefrom.

The uric-acid purines that meat contains are very strong irritants, but such continuous excitation of the nerves, as Dr. Ralph Bircher of the Bircher-Benner Clinic notes, is no road to strength.

Says Dr. Bircher:

In athletics, the last degree of performance must be extracted. Where regeneration and recovery demand detoxification and metabolic economy, the advantages of a meatless diet show up with special clarity. Despite meat's reputation as a source of well-balanced amino acids, tests show on the contrary that 5 to 10 times as much tryptophane and 5 to 7 times as much tyrosine are found in the dry substances of meat as are found in vegetable protein sources. . . .

Meat also contains excessive amounts of the amino acid methionine, which, according to investigations at Harvard, were shown to favor hardening of the arteries. (Charcoal broil that steak and you add the carcinogenic properties of six hundred cigarettes!)

Meat is notoriously low in calcium. A negative calcium balance can lead to osteoporosis, which can put an end to your career as a duffer or diver in pretty short order, and this can most often be traced to years of heavy meat eating. A condition called arthrosis occurs, and athletes who eat much meat are especially susceptible to arthrosis. According the The British Medical Journal, *The Lancet,* "Among 20 professional soccer players who were observed for 18 years, there was 100% incidence of ankle and 97.5% incidence of knee arthrosis."

Meat is harder to digest than other more or equally proteinaceous foods, too. According to J. H. Kellogg in *The New Dietetics,* even moderate meat eaters require of their kidneys three times the amount of work in the elimination of nitrogeneous wastes than is demanded of the kidneys of flesh abstainers.

High meat diets raise the cholesterol levels, thereby offsetting to a certain extent the cholesterol-lowering effects of a high-exercise regime. Experiments by the Department of Nutrition at Loma Linda University in

California show that a diet high in legumes such as chick peas reduces cholesterol levels. Meat, on the other hand, with its large amounts of cholesterol and saturated fats, was found to stimulate the body's production of this villainous stuff.

Meat, in contrast to roughage foods like raw carrots, leafy greens, and whole grains, contains little fiber and so gives the organs of elimination too little to do. And impacted bowels at match point are no better than a clogged artery on the fifty-yard line.

Meat is a poor match for the complete protein that comes from combining certain grains, grits, greens, and nuts. Just a bit of miso, an agreeably salty soybean paste, spread on whole-grain bread supplies five times more protein than a "quarter pounder," according to writer Bill Shurtleff, co-author of *The Book of Miso*.

Furthermore, "We have never seen a new vegetarian who was overweight," writes Darla Erhard, a research nutritionist at San Francisco General Hospital.

Meat is low in carbohydrate, ergo a poor source for go power. "The inhabitants of Ecuador and the primitive Hunzas in India are either complete or almost complete vegetarians," according to biochemist Paavo Airola. "They eat a high-carbohydrate low-protein diet, and their strength is phenomenal. They run for two days at a time."

"Meat," adds Dr. E. V. McCollum, Johns Hopkins University professor, "is not essential for endurance. This has been demonstrated by whole races and certain individuals more than once." And the formidably named and formidably accomplished English Vegetarian Cycling and Athletics Club has certainly demonstrated that such a diet does it, more than once. At one time, this club held 40 percent of the national cycling road records, and their members range in age from early twenties to late seventies.

As writer Karen Cross Whyte points out in her recent book, *The Original Diet,*

> In general, primates are meat eaters by rare accident, from about 150 million years ago until the emergence of man about 5 million years ago early primates were overwhelmingly vegetarian . . . 99% of that time all food was eaten raw and in its natural state. . . . The very high civilizations of the Aztecs, Incas and Mayas flourished on a diet that was 80% to 90% vegetable food. . . .

Another of meat's negative characteristics is the presence of a substance called siderophilic protein material, which is similar to the phytates in grains, the oxalates in vegetables, and the carbonates in other foods. These substances do their dirty work by binding up the naturally occurring iron in the food and preventing its absorption. This interference with the absorption of dietary iron coming from what is generally considered our foremost source of iron is quite ironic as well as quite worrisome since it causes a great deal of what is called "sports anemia," according to Professor Kvanta of Sweden.[9]

If you don't give a fig for carrots, celery, and leafy greens, where does that leave you? Is a diet free or nearly free of burgers, steaks, and stews likely to be a lemon or a lifesaver for you?

Certainly vegetarian foods are, no bones about it, energizing.

In another study, [10] for instance, the celebrated Per-Olaf Astrand conducted aseries of experiments to determine the best diet for athletes. He administered a mixed diet of protein, fat, and carbohydrate to his subjects. They then pedaled one hour and fifty-four minutes before dropping from exhaustion. He then administered a diet high in fat and protein (including meat) to the same subjects, who tired after fifty-seven minutes this time. And finally, on a diet of carbohydrate-rich fruits, cereals and vegetables (excluding meat) the subjects cycled for two hours and forty-seven minutes before stopping. Some of them even continued for an additional two hours.

Another study that came up with similar results was conducted by Dr. Irving Fisher of Yale University to test the differences in stamina of vegetarians versus meat eaters. Dr. Fisher found that few of the meat eaters were able to hold their arms horizontal for more than 15 minutes. By contrast, the vegetarians were able to hold their arms in that position for better than an hour, experiencing little pain or discomfort. One member of the vegetarian group managed to stand spread-eagled for three hours and twenty minutes before calling it quits. In a subsequent test, the vegetarians again beat out the meat eaters in the number of knee bends completed without pain or discomfort. The score: meat eaters 300 to 400 with side effects, including pain and weakness in the thigh muscles. Vegetarians scored 1,800 to 5,000 knee bends and no reported soreness.[11]

"A vegetarian diet causes men to run faster and longer," observed a Los Angeles News commentator covering the remarkable occasion in 1976 when the record for the world's marathon was shattered by a seven-man twenty-four-hour relay team, all of them vegetarians. The team was led by forty-five-year old David Park, M.D. Other team members ranged in age from twenty-three to thirty-eight years old.

And then there are such vegetable-powered athletes as racing cyclists Franz S. Dusika (age sixty) and Max Bulla (age sixty-three), who in 1968 cycled nonstop the entire round-trip distance from Vienna to Barcelona to Casbah-Tunis-Rome to Vienna, a total of 3,420 miles at a clip of 110 miles a day for an average riding speed of 18 miles per hour.

Finally, consider the incredible Hulda Crooks, the

eighty-seven-year-old vegetarian dietitian who has climbed Mt. Whitney thirteen times.

It is obvious that meat is an expendable element in any eating-to-win diet. What, then, is at stake if you decide to drop steak? Very little. In fact, the meat totalers diet seems to be a boon to the brain and the blood stream as well, according to two recent studies. The first, reported in the *Journal of the American Dietetic Association,* revealed that nondairy-consuming vegetarians (also known as vegans) had more red blood cells per cubic centimeter than any other group studied. This is, of course, crucial to oxygen transmission by the blood and also was interpreted as meaning that vegans (who abstain from eggs and milk as well as meat) are getting the greatest flow of oxygenated blood to their brain cells.

The second study, at Stanford University, indicated that vegetarians had higher levels of blood ascorbic acid than meat eaters. Ascorbic acid, which plays an important role in the neurochemical electrical signals in the brain's circuitry, is prevalent in fruits and vegetables but absent in all but raw, undoctored meats.

A diet rich in fresh vegetables and vegetable oils is one of the primary factors involved in promoting "good cholesterol" reported both *The Herbalist* and *Time* magazines in the fall of 1977.

Not only are they fiber foods, the reports note, but they contain those nutrients essential to building HDL (high-density lipoproteins) levels in the body. Lipoproteins not only carry off cholesterol but may actually help flush away fatty deposits from plaque on arterial walls.

Also on the plus side, vegetarianism can greatly improve your cholesterol levels, and lowered blood fat levels have certainly been known to spruce up sagging sprint times and soccer scores. It can also improve (i.e., lower) your triglyceride levels.

According to Dr. Donald Monkerud, writing in a 1976

issue of *Runners World Magazine,* "A high-fat high-cholesterol diet leads to closure of the arteries, and no amount of running will fully re-open the arteries once they're clogged." But the good news, confirmed by M.D.-marathoner Joan Ullyot in her book *Women's Running,* is that vegetarian runners have the lowest cholesterol and triglyceride readings of all groups studied, followed by meat-eating runners, then by nonrunning vegetarians.

Obviously, it's a combination of diet and exercise that does it. Neither one does the trick without the other.

For instance, famous French racing cyclists Fausto Coppi and Luis Ocana were food doctored to victory by the author-herbalist Maurice Messague on a strict routine of raw fruits, vegetables, and whole grains and honey. A similar diet worked for superswimmer Murray Rose, the youngest triple Olympic Gold medalist in the 1950s. Rose, a vegetarian from birth, ate a diet rich in nuts, seeds, whole grains, fruits, vegetables, and goat's milk.

Similarly, Johnny Weismuller and Bill Walton only hit their strides after switching to meat-free diets. Other vegetarians who are loaded for bear include Amby Burfoot, winner of the 1968 Boston Marathon, and six of the top ten finishers at the 1970 World Veterans Marathon in Germany.

Some of the greatest marathon runners in the world are the Tarahumara Indians of northwestern Mexico, who run kickball races that sometimes last two days and two nights and cover 200 miles. Their diet—except for an occasional bit of goat meat—is a high-carbohydrate, low-protein vegetarian diet.

The tide may be turning against steak and spuds even in the body building field, long notorious for its emphasis on high-meat diets. Vince Gerondi, the physical-culture chieftain who has trained more Mr. Americas than any other body builder in the world, recently spoke out against the practice of "pumping protein." He was quoted in

Vegetarian World: "A negative nitrogen balance is cata-
bolic, leads to gout, sluggishness, liver and kidney problems, and toxemia, among other things." Gerondi's own
diet emphasizes a lot of fertile raw eggs, raw milk, and
cheese and no more than 45 grams of protein a day. In
addition, Gerondi advocates a protein fast one day a
week, eating just vegetables to pump sodium back into the
liver.

In common with the world's most famous trainer of
runners, Ernst Van Aaken, Gerondi goes overboard for
undereating, something that is more easily accomplished
on a diet that excludes meat.

And just as a bonus, should you need a bit more
incentive to keep you away from hamburger heaven, it
seems that "just vegetating," can bring a certain measure
of protection against cancer. Which may have nothing
directly to do with your next crosscourt volley but is of
paramount importance in whether you play at all. The
research of Dr. Tsuneo Kada, a mutation specialist at the
National Institute of Genetics in Japan, has demonstrated
that certain vegetables, among them cabbage, turnips,
asparagus, and bean sprouts, have the ability to deactivate
cancer-causing substances in the body.[12]

For Dick Gregory, conversion to a noncarnivorous
mode of eating came in a finger-lickin' flash. "Wouldn't it
be wild if (we) found out that God was a chicken? I just
hope that if that ever happens, I'm standing there right
behind Colonel Sanders. I'd whisper in his ear, 'Go on and
tell Chicken Big he's finger-lickin' good.'"

For Gregory, it is not just vegetarianism that does it but
a diet of totally raw vegetarian foods—vegetarianism plus,
as it were.

Gregory now has moved on to an even more radical
mode, becoming one of the supporters of fruitarianism,
which concentrates on fruits, with vegetables and nuts
thrown in.

No-meat diets like the frugavorian one may be a boon to some but is bad news indeed for even more athletes, according to British physician Dr. Constance Leslie. In the course of researching the effects of pectin on lowering blood cholesterol levels, she put herself on an all-fruit diet. Her cholesterol came down, and Dr. Leslie herself came down with anemia and a number of other malnutritional disorders.

Such extremes aside, it isn't difficult to round up playing-field testimony that a lot of steak gnoshing can make you sluggish.

Vegetarianism may cost you nothing but the blessed loss of that all too occasional "overstuffed" feeling. As tennist Harold Solomon moaned to an interviewer in *Tennis Magazine,* "Steak takes a lot of time to digest. Carbohydrates are almost instantly converted to energy." Solomon had just lost his match to an unseeded player thirty minutes after a steak dinner.

Worries about adequate protein intake on a meatless diet are unfounded. According to Britain's *Lancet,*

Formerly, vegetable proteins were classified as second class and regarded as inferior to first-class proteins of animal origin. But this distinction has now been largely discarded. Many field studies have shown that the proteins provided by suitable mixtures of vegetables enable children to grow no less well than children provided with milk and other animal proteins.

Vegetarians can be well nourished and then some, says Roger J. Williams, author of *Nutrition in a Nutshell,* "if they eat wisely and include leaves, seeds, roots, and fruit in their diets."

Inside every soybean there's more power than in a Big Mac. Try a vegetable diet. You just might like it, and vice versa.

Raw-food Vegetarianism

You can always get a second wind, but you can't take out a second mortgage on your liver or your kidneys, so don't overwork them with too much protein. That's hard to do on a diet that passes up cooked foods entirely. As a raw-foods vegetarian, you should experience boundless energy, say the diet's advocates. But will you get enough to eat, enough body-building protein?

"It is practically impossible," says Paavo Airola, "to eat a natural food without eating some protein." And Dr. Eimer's studies in Germany also deflate any fears of protein deficiency. Athletes who changed from a diet containing 100 grams of animal protein to one supplying only 50 grams of protein from vegetarian sources continued to perform with no change on the down side. Indeed, their records in some cases even improved.

And why not? It is a well-established fact that acidosis and fatigue are likely to occur as a side effect of high-protein loading with meat. Complex carbohydrates burn "clean," while the fats in proteins such as meat and dairy products burn only 85-90 percent, and the residue remains as an acid pileup of ketones. Bad.

Objections to a diet that not only excludes meat but eliminates cooked food as well are neatly countered by raw foodist Karen Cross Whyte, who tells us, "No animal other than man has ever cooked its food. Raw foods are the most natural for all animals, including man." And she adds further fuel to the unfired food controversy by quoting British anthropologist Edmund Leach:

> It isn't a biological necessity that you should cook your food. It is a custom, a symbolic act, a piece of magic that transforms the substance and removes the contamination of 'otherness.' ... Raw food is dirty and dangerous; cooked food is clean and safe ... the

cooking of food is both an assertion of this otherness and a means of getting rid of anxiety which otherness generates. . . ." [13]

The epitome of raw foodism is probably the Waerland Natural Foods Diet, developed over twenty years ago by the "unusually energetic and brilliant scholar of Swedish descent, Are Waerland," as he was described by the authors of *The Runners Diet.* This diet itself is

only part of a biologically correct system of living which includes plenty of fresh air, sunshine, and aerobic exercise. It also involves avoiding all table and cooking salt, coffee, strong tea, meat, fish and eggs, drinking at meals, very hot drinks any time, tobacco, alcohol, sweets, chocolate, white bread and cakes made of white flour.

Tough as all this sounds, it has its fans in the stands and on the blocks.

If it isn't as simple a discipline as fasting, raw foodism comes close. It will certainly save you considerable time and money if you stop cooking and partaking of the cow and its fellows. Your overall protein intake can be reduced when all your protein is coming from nonmeat sources. Thanks to its high enzyme content, raw food digests itself.

Anyway, eating lots of cooked protein causes lots of problems. Proteins are altered by heat to unassimilable forms, says endocrinologist and author Henry Bieler.[14] If, for instance, the amino acid lysine is damaged, the body may be totally unable to handle the other amino acids you're taking in. T-bone steak may not be providing you with "balanced protein" at all, in other words.

According to Creig Hoyt, [15] recent evidence points to some of the minor breakdown products of cooked protein as direct inhibitors of brain and muscle function.

Raw foods are quite probably the ingredients of the ideal diet for the dedicated idealistic athlete, says the editor of *Sportsmedicine.* "The diet conforms to the description of the perfect pre-game repast. The diet in the 48 hours preceding sports competition should be high in carbohydrates, moderate in fat content and relatively low in protein." [16]

According to Dr. Bircher-Benner, one of the pioneers in nutrition before the discovery of vitamins and enzymes, raw foods contain a higher order and quality of nutritive energy plus life-sustaining and curative powers. These ideas were confirmed forty years later by Dublin's Nobel Prize-winning physicist Schroedinger and the University of Vienna's Eppinger.

Dr. John M. Douglass developed this hypothesis: "Since early man lived entirely on raw food, perhaps such a diet would be less stressful to the human system in general and less likely to produce diabetes than a cooked diet."

After testing his hunch, he was able to report in the *Annals of Internal Medicine* that when his diabetic patients ate a diet consisting of 90–100 percent raw food, they were able to completely discontinue medication. Another study also found that such a diet allowed for a considerable reduction in the amount of insulin necessary. Maybe on a raw foods diet you too will begin to "cook."

Fat Loading

If your energy levels are in arrears, there is "fat loading," although nobody calls it that. After all, you get more energy gram for gram from fats than from any other food group.

Why do fats have such a high energy yield? Because they have a low oxygen content. On a weight basis, fats yield two and a half times as many calories as carbohydrates.

Dr. Joan Ullyot, one of our foremost fat backers and

fat-fact finders, is a physiology researcher and a thin acclimatized marathon runner. She explains that "there is a difference between 'trained-on fat' and 'eaten-on fat'.... Much of the body's fat—especially that stored by trained long-distance runners—is highly active metabolically and serves as a superior fuel for endurance performance ... this kind of fat has a much higher yield per gram than glycogen, and is easily stored in the nooks and crannies of the body. . . ."

And something else: The heart burns fat in preference to all other fuels.

Fats are the carriers of the fat-soluble vitamins (A, D, E, K), and they have a satiety value other foods don't provide due to their very slow transit time through the stomach and small intestine.

It could be that you are a mountain climber with an aversion to fat. What then?

According to Dr. Gene W. Mason,[17] "At high altitudes people tolerate carbohydrates better. You get twice as many calories out of fat as you do from carbohydrates, but many people don't tolerate it well. For those who can tolerate fatty foods it is their advantage to eat them."

"The leading role given carbohydrates in recent years should be very much de-emphasized," says Ernst Van Aaken.[18] "All the carbohydrates you could possibly store would only last you 18.7 miles of a marathon at most." Van Aaken believes that stored adipose fat is a much better source of fuel than glycogen since it has a much higher energy per gram.

If you burn a higher percentage of fat (and the better trained you are, the more fat you'll burn) your glycogen stores last longer. Not that Dr. Van Aaken believes that fat loading is the answer for us all, either. "No more than 40 grams of fat should be eaten, including 15 grams of butter and 25 grams of oils rich in linoleic acid."

In general, men burn more carbohydrates in exercise,

says Van Aaken, while women burn a relatively higher amount of the fatty acids and maybe cholesterol, too. He speculates that the female system may be better geared to metabolize fat.

And if you are going to explore the advantages of a higher fat diet for sport, couple it with some B_{15}. B_{15}-rich foods seem to improve fat metabolism.

Point two, if you plan to try fat-loading or to increase the fat content in your diet for performance sake, is to add sufficient amounts of biotin, choline, inositol and lecithin rich foods to your meals. An insufficiency of any of these B vitamins in the presence of increased dietary fat resulted in fat-loaded livers and vascular systems at least when the eaters were rats, according to a report by Paul De Kruif cited by the January 1978 issue of *Bestways* magazine. It is believed that the human system runs the same risks without those three B vitamins and lecithin, all of which work as a team in metabolizing fats.

Both Dr. Robert C. Atkins and trainer Per-Olaf Astrand consider fat the main fuel supply in light exercise, which produces a pulse rate under 120.

What about an ultra fat diet for energy? How much fat can your body handle without experiencing problems?

If you are anything like explorer-anthropologist Vilhjalmur Steffansson, you may benefit by the "Stone Age Diet." This diet consists of large amounts of meat, heavy cream, and other foods that are high in natural fats. No margarine and no sugar or processed foods. Given a trial run in 1959 by Steffansson and his wife, butter, bacon, and even suet were included, but anything refined or processed, and all empty calories were totally eliminated. No starchy vegetables were eaten, either.

The result? Steffansson found he had twice the energy of most men of fifty; he could work ten to twelve hours a day; his blood pressure normalized, and his cholesterol dropped. His arthritis disappeared, and he lost 17 pounds.

Steffansson's experiment, of much earlier vintage (1928), under the medical supervision of the diabetic ward of Bellevue Hospital in New York, in partnership with fellow explorer Karsten Anderson, also proved that fats bear fruit. But that time the emphasis was on meat, ruling out dairy products. After a year on this seemingly bizarre one-food-group diet, "Both Anderson and Steffansson were in better health than at its start. . . ." [19]

So maybe if you're chock full of nuts, butter, and eggs, you stand a fat chance of getting there first.

Fasting

Another diet, based on the idea that you are what you did eat but don't anymore, is fasting.

Will fasting make you faster? It certainly puts wings on some feet. In England a man named Park Barner ran a double marathon on a stomach that had not been filled for twenty-four hours, and he finished it a half hour sooner than the doubler he'd done previously.

Runners World Magazine tells how, in 1964, a team of Swedish walkers hiked for a fortnight. They covered 300 miles, eating nothing and dropping an average of 15 pounds each of stored energy. Says M.D.-marathoner George Sheehan, "There is a time for meat, a time for bread, and a time for nothing at all. The problem is finding the right time."

One group of athletes that doesn't have trouble finding the right time are the athletes surveyed by a runners' magazine in 1975. Some 13 percent of them said they frequently fasted for one to three days before a race, taking only water and juices.

Ian Jackson, editor of *Soccer World,* is also a water-and-juice faster. He sustains himself on these for a week at a time, during which he logs 20 or more miles of running a day.

Why? Because as author Herbert Shelton, considered

the first man of fasting by some, says, "Digestion is real work. To cease eating for a time constitutes one of the surest means of rest." [20]

And as another trainer-runner observed in print, "The body runs on . . . the reserves it has built up in months and years of long training, chiefly in the liver, musculature and hormones, as well as in the enzymes. Digestion shortly before or after a race wastes energy. . . ."

Fasting should be of special interest to any athlete who is trying to peak because it gives the digestive system a chance to switch off, thus releasing lots of energy for other purposes.

As one fasting spokesman put it, "The fasting organism nourishes its functioning tissues upon intrinsic nutrient stores and removes all accumulated and stored debris from its precincts."

German running coach Ernst Van Aaken, M.D., says you should be able to live off your own resources for long periods if you are moderately healthy. Even runners in ultramarathons (50 miles or more) are often advised to fast twelve to twenty-four hours prior to competition.

Why? Because most trouble that marathoners encounter at the 20-mile mark is due to "the body's never having been forced to learn to switch over to conversion of stored fats after it runs out of glycogen," according to Van Aaken.

He's talking about fasting, the discipline by which the body learns that valuable trick.

And what happens when the body switches over? The body switches over to fat metabolism for energy. This happens, Van Aaken says,

in trained marathon runners usually at about 30–32 kilometers, where the runner must persevere until the body has begun to deliver sugar from the body's fat deposits which the organism is able to convert into sugar. Runs of 100 kilos and walks of over 500 kilos use up the entire stored carbohydrates in a few hours. These runners and walkers nevertheless survive, even running better, if they've fasted for a day before the race.

You can teach your body to shift gears if you train when you are hungry or work out at least fourteen hours after eating. Then the body learns to use fats and carbohydrates for energy.

There are minuses associated with fasting, though. It can lead to potassium deficiency, for one thing, and that loss in turn causes muscular weakness and other dysfunctions, putting the player at a distinct disadvantage.

Also, sodium deficiency may be a result and on its heels fatigue since it affects the adrenal glands and lowers blood pressure. According to the Congress of Clinical Application of Zinc Metabolism (Cleveland, 1971), you stand to lose as much as 15 percent of your body's store of zinc, too.

Other negative possibilities include impaired kidney function and respiratory problems.

If you are very thin, you are on the list of sports species endangered by fasting. But fasting usually works like a charm for the overweight, since extra poundage is a guard against an excessive loss of protein.

Dr. Alan Cott, author of two books on fasting, is reassuring: "Fasting normalizes the metabolism. The kidneys preserve potassium and sugar in the blood—important elements that assure our feeling of well being."

Dr. Alex Carrel in *Man the Unknown* lends support to this view. "The proteins of the muscles and the glands are mobilized, all the organs sacrifice their own substances in order to maintain blood, heart and brain in a normal condition. Fasting purifies and profoundly modifies our tissues."

But still, in the initial stages of a fast 75 grams of protein are lost each day, although this decreases in time to 18–24 grams. How can you keep your strength up if you're putting nothing down? Well, you could cheat a little. Two Swedish scientists, Carlstrom and Rooth, consider it important for the faster to have small amounts of protein during the fast.

Such semi-fasting is not such a bad idea, thinks Dr. Alex Comfort of London's University College, who has increased the life span of rats 50 percent just by feeding them two days out of three.

Fans of fasting say it is a painless way to drop pounds, to increase energy, and provide a kind of hormonal high similar to the euphoria long-distance runners experience. The late tennis-playing author, Paul C. Bragg, said fasting made him feel "like a human dynamo." At eighty-five he was still fasting in stretches of twenty-four to thirty-six hours once a week.

As for the mechanics, compared to carbohydrate loading and other eating-to-win plans requiring charts, diaries, and commercial elixirs, fasting is simplicity itself. It requires no weighing in, no stocking up, and no counting out.

But check with your doctor before you do anything. You may be one of the special cases for whom fasting is a not a go-go but a no-no.

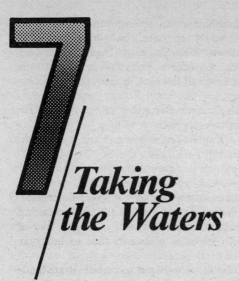

7/ Taking the Waters

Got the hots? Sure. Everybody who exercises gets them. But the question is how best to satify your thirst out there on the playing field. With a short beer, a long drink of water, a sip of soda, or a can of juice?

You are sweating away large amounts of essential minerals and chemicals known as electrolytes (sodium, potassium, iron, magnesium) and these, along with fluid, protect you from dehydration's devastating effects, which include everything from plain thirst to impaired vision, heat stroke, and brain damage.

There are an incredible number of choices. Even the choices have choices. If for instance, you have virtuously decided to quench your thirst with nothing but natural water, you still have to decide what kind of water.

There is, for instance, distilled water, but that's devoid

of minerals. There's sparkling spring water, but that may be too costly. There's tap water, but chances are that's contamined with something or is too high in potentially toxic metal like copper and too low in zinc, another essential mineral. And tap water, in the opinion of Swiss cellular therapist Dr. Benjamin Frank, "usually contains fluorides, which have a damaging effect on oxidative metabolism and energy production."

Trainer Ernst Van Aaken advises, "It is a mistake to drink too much water, thinning the body's salt supplies while ... eliminating concentrated salt solution through sweat. ..."

You and the sedentary man in the street are uniquely different when it comes to the matter of fluid replacement. While he might metabolize 2.5 liters of liquid daily, the figure for you, if you are a real endurance athlete, might be as high as 4–5 liters, and falling somewhere in between if your sport is one of light to moderate intensity, for example, tennis, cycling, etc.

Water is necessary for all energy production, for temperature controls, for elimination of the by-products of cell metabolism. Participation in even moderate exercise demands a minimum of 32 ounces of fluid for every 1,000 calories of food ingested if you are exercising. To put it another way, the body requires 7–14 ounces of water for every thirty minutes of strenuous exercise.

"On hot, humid days," advises Dr. Robert Leach, "players should literally replace their fluid loss as it is being lost. Fluid loss is cumulative. With a loss of three pounds, there is a decrease in endurance and possibly motor coordination. With 5 pounds of weight loss, the player must force fluids to regain this weight within a 24-hour period."

The problem, continues Dr. Leach, is that "heat fatigue may happen to anyone and is not related to physical conditioning but to acclimatization to hot humid weather.

High humdity decreases the effectiveness of sweating to cool the body and thus increases the heat stroke possibilities."

The danger of heat stroke and heat exhaustion, too often the result of a potassium-poor diet, should not be underestimated. Each year even young athletes die or suffer as a result of one and the other.

Heat exhaustion sets in when the body is having trouble coping with heat but still manages by various means, including sweating, to keep the core temperature near normal.

Heat stroke, on the other hand, occurs when the body can no longer deal with heat. There is a rapid rise in temperature to 106, which may be the prelude to death.

You, like most athletes, probably are underhydrated. If you're not a faithful water drinker, you can replace liquid loss with foods that are specially juicy, such as tomatoes, oranges, and watermelon and tangerines.

Hydration is important even when you are not over-heated. Eight glasses of liquid a day would not be out of line. But the temperature of the liquid is important, too. Ice-cold water is always a no-no because it chills the digestive machinery. Physician Charlotte Holmes says everyone should follow a water-drinking program, beginning with at least two glasses of water upon arising and followed by subsequent glasses spaced throughout the day.[1]

There are times to suspend water as well. Washing a meal down with water is verboten because it dilutes the important stomach acids that digest foods.

An alternative is to eat fruit at the start of a meal to satisfy thirst, to drink an hour before meals, or to drink a "nonwater" like buttermilk, which isn't a liquid but a food since it turns into curds when it hits the stomach and encounters the stomach's acids.

The notion that a cold beer on a hot day is just what the

doctor ordered can brew trouble, too, since a single beer can lower your heat tolerance for as long as three days.

Anyway, look what else one brew can do to you. According to studies at the University of California at Berkeley, the alcohol in even one drink can cause temporary but important changes in vision. The ability to see fine details after exposure to bright light also deteriorates, and recovery from glare takes up to 50 percent longer, bad news no matter what your sport.[2]

In addition, beer may contain a number of artificial ingredients that don't improve anybody's game, such as propylene glycol, alginate, sodium bisulfite, qualsia extract, calcium disodium EDTA. And there are two food colorings allowed in beer: blue number one and yellow number five.

Modern brewing technology destroys every dietary property in beer except one: calories. Beer is not the liquid bread it used to be. They've taken the yeast out of it, so all those beneficial B complex vitamins are long gone. Most popular brews, says the *Vegetarian Review,* are loaded with malt sugar, another refined product that contributes little to nutritional needs. There's no telling what a bottle of beer has in it: Beer is not only exempt from the laws requiring detailed ingredient labeling, it need not even disclose the amount of alcohol contained.

As for wine, there are seventy or more chemical additives dumped in it, say Gary and Steve Null. Asbestos, an infamous carcinogenic agent, is used in most popular wines as a filtering agent.

Alcohol in all forms is a diuretic that irritates the kidneys and causes them to excrete more water. Roy Ald says, "Adding alcohol to the diet is ridiculous, and anyone performing vigorous exercise should know that ... alcoholic beverages constrict the arteries leading to the heart. When you are exerting yourself, the heart demands a greatly accelerated blood flow. The result can be disastrous, and that goes for any vigorous acitvity. The runner, for instance, who had a few drinks should allow an interval of at least two and a half hours to pass before he takes a workout."

If you really want a drink to undo all your training efforts take coffee. Coffee raises the blood sugar temporarily and then drops it down to dangerously low levels that cause an oxygen deficiency in the heart muscle. In addition, it may interfere with iron absorption and result in a shortage of inositol, another B vitamin that is also involved in proper heart-muscle functioning. Coffee also increases cholesterol and fat levels in the blood.

"Caffeine" says sports writer Robert Wieder, "a stimulant which is as bad for your body as any third rail, is also taken in concentrated tablets and 250 mg. shots. Though a popular lab poison and addicting over a period of time, caffeine has been banned by nobody and is a special hit with Eastern European jocks. Strongly linked to heart trouble, it is also—along with cocaine and strychnine—routinely used to quell fatigue."

Caffeine in coffee stimulates the heart, brain, and nervous system and thus contributes to your stress debit. According to a study by the California State University in Los Angeles of the caffeine content of coffees, "dripolated" coffee is the most potent of all, followed by percolated coffee and then drip and instant. Drip coffee is usually twice as strong as instant. Swiss researchers discovered that after drinking one quart of coffee much of the body's B_1 had been obliterated. The offender was not caffeine this time. It was the chlorogenic acid that coffee contains. And coffee also uses up another B vitamin, biotin, and a biotin deficiency weakens both the heart and the lungs.

Then there is the trouble with tea. According to studies by the Society for Experimental Biology, four to six cups of tea, even when taken as part of a nutritionally adequate diet, induce B_1 deficiency. And you know how important B_1 is in making the proper energy connections. Within a week after being on the tea-drinking regimen, all the volunteers showed B_1 deficiencies, which in some cases were classified as severe. The hypothesis is that there is a chemical union of the vitamin to the tannin in tea that makes the vitamin unavailable.[3]

And another wetting solution that will leave you high and dry is soda, the primary ought-nought that is discussed in Junk Foods.

Sodas have been cited for their ability to do everything from eroding the teeth to generating cancerous tumors. Most soft drinks contain brominated vegetable oil (BVO), and some research suggests that over a short period of time BVO ingredients can damage the liver, heart, kidney and spleen. Many sodas also contain caffeine, which causes fluctuations in blood-sugar levels, especially harmful to the hypoglycemic athlete.

Caffeinated soft drinks also irritate the digestive tract, interfere with the action of enzymes, and together with tannin, which may also be a part of your favorite soft brew, is suspected as a weak carcinogen. There may also be bisulfite lurking within, a chemical that brought about genetic damage in tests with lab animals, or carbonic acid, which has been found to damage the tissues in the eye. The water used may be contaminated or fluoridated. And soft drinks are highly acidic, too.

According to *Diabetes Magazine,* "A can of carbonated soda which can be swallowed in a minute or two, contains 38 grams of sugar. To obtain this amount of sugar from food one would have to eat four apples, four pears, 7 ounces of bananas, or 10 ounces of plums."

Optional ingredients that need not be on a soda can's label include any one of twelve nutritive sweeteners, eight acidifying agents, thirty-two buffering agents, seventeen emulsifiers, six foaming agents, and one antifoaming agent.

Soda replacements include carrot juice, which is good for the liver, and green juices, which help the pancreas, from beet greens, lettuce, cabbage, comfrey leaves, celery, and cucumber.

Vegetable juices are the builders of the body, while fruit juices (which do not combine well with vegetables) are the body's cleansers. If you have a blender or juicer, there are more ways of producing a rejuvenating juice than Pepsi has plants. And they *are* the real thing. According to runner-mountainclimber Thorwald Boie, author of *The Raw Food Diet Plan,* a good raw food diet can overcome most of the discomforts and dangers of dehydration, especially in hot weather. The best drink of all, in his estimation, may be the one you can sink your teeth into. "Raw fruits," says Boie, "such as mangoes, pineapples, bananas, coconuts are excellent humid-day foods and contain water in its best form, easy to digest and not overtaxing to the body."

So what should your cup runneth over with on a hot day?

Orange juice has a lot of things going for it. Michael Jacobsen gives it top marks.

But all juices are not created equal. Some can considerably cramp your style nutritionally. "With a real-juice product," says Consumer's Union in rating the orange-drink mixes, you won't be pouring your morning pick-me-up from a chemists flask." Orange-drink mixes are by and large very poor imitations of the real thing. They are high in sodium (14–29 mg. per six-ounce portion compared to 2½ mg. in fresh juice) and low in potassium (a 6-ounce glass of real juice provides 2.34 mg, whereas an equal amount of Tang provides only .52 mg). The survey also pointed out that in most brands of powdered juice, nutrients added for purposes of fortification only supplied as little as 10 percent of the RDA.

A recent study of the vitamin value of other kinds of processed orange juice casts considerable doubt on the assumption that they are equal to the fresh orange itself. As reported in the *Journal of the American Medical Association,* frozen juice and especially carton juice tended to have a very significant portion of its vitamin C in the oxidated form, which has no nutritional value.

What's more, reconstituted juice concentrate in cartons, as *Prevention Magazine* points out, is "cooked down and pasteurized, so it will stay fresh longer. Ascorbic acid, however, does not usually go through such processing intact."

For what the real McCoy offers you, see the chart in Appendix II.

Are commerical "isotonic" or "synthetic sweat drinks" the solution? The virtue of such commercial "ades" or "synthetic sweat" solutions is that they are a simulation of the extracellular body fluids that contain water, salts, and glucose. Supposedly, they are absorbed twelve times faster than water.

One of the shortcomings of the commercial "ade" drinks is that although they give you the electrolytes you're losing, they may not be giving you enough of them. They seem to work best if they are there in sweatlike proportions.

How much salt are you shedding when you sweat? Experts say .2–.5 of your perspiration is salt. Adding salt to your drink may offset some of this loss. It will also lengthen the time the drink spends in your stomach.

But the more salt you take in, the more potassium you'll lose, and according to *Medical Times,* more heat strokes are actually the result of potassium, not sodium, shortages.

If you are an unacclimatized athlete, Dr. Martin Eisman warns that synthetic sweat drinks won't do you much good because they cannot replace what you lose fast enough. Many of them don't have any more potassium or sodium than a glass of orange juice or a mug of milk. And many neglect to add any magnesium at all.

Probably the ideal hydration for a moderately active athlete would be one Dr. Arthur Mollen of Phoenix, himself a marathoner, has postulated: a three-stage electrolyte glucose drink. But until that becomes available, you'd be better off with homemade hydrations that are simple solutions minus the refined sugars, salts, and additional chemicals that commercial electrolyte replacement drinks often contain. According to Ernst Van Aaken, "Even so-called athletic drinks, used in cycle racing tours and running distances of marathon and greater length, serve no purpose of giving the body nutritional elements and calories. They only permit the utilization of body reserves, especially fat and glycogen. . . ." [4]

Whatever kind of hydration you home-make to pour down your hatch, remember to go easy on the sugar. Sugar upsets blood-sugar levels, interferes with digestion and energy production, dissipates important water-soluble B vitamins, and, like salt, gets into the circulation too fast and out of the stomach too slowly. "Sugar concentration of any drink intended as a replacement fluid should not exceed 2½ percent," warns Peter Van Handel of the Human Performance Laboratories. He adds that the effectiveness of alternative sweeteners (such as honcy) to combat fatigue seems to depend on their concentration in the solution.

For a few hydrators to whip up in your own kitchen, see Appendix I.

8 / The Energy Connection, Part 1

Calories and the Athletic Body

"The slender figure of Harold Norpoth or Filbert Bayi, among other world-class distance runners, is considered suspect by many people. But what *is* healthy if 13:20 for 5,000 meters or 3:32 for 1,500 meters isn't?" asks Ernst Van Aaken.

This phenomenon of looking bad, too thin by the nonathlete's standards, yet performing good by anybody's standards is often one of the "training effects" of several months of ardent running, a sport that has a higher-than-average quota of skinny-minnies.

That's no surprise, since shaking your bootee at a rate of 6–7 miles an hour is defined by Britain's *Athletic Weekly* as the mode in which oxygen is being used up at the rate of 800 calories an hour, with glycogen expenditure of 200 grams an hour.

A survey at Olympic Village Cafeteria in Montreal in 1977 revealed that the average caloric intake for participating athletes was 5,500 daily.

How many calories should you take in to compensate for the energy you're expending in tennis, swimming, running, cycling, and so on?

The ultimate calorie users are sprinters and high jumpers. The latter burn 100,000 calories an hour, but only for a fraction of a second; the former use 10,000, but only for a few seconds. Marathon runners use roughly 900 calories an hour for over two hours, and long-distance walkers may burn up 350 calories an hour for days at a time.

The answer to how large a calorie intake depends on the athlete and the event. Swimmer Diana Nyad, for instance, preps herself this way:

"I drink a hot powdered liquid that provides me with 1300 calories. In a race, my blood sugar drops below metabolism level in three minutes. A cup of this stuff every hour barely helps."

Some nutritional writers and trainers cover their bets by giving you considerable margin—somewhere between 3,500 and 6,500 calories, they say, for the somewhat-to-the-truly active lay athlete, taking sex, size, sport, and age into consideration, too.

"Long-distance runners," says nutritionist Dr. Jean Mayer, "require more calories a day than any other group." And no group agrees with him more than the runners themselves.

Other experts, however, do not. "The way runners eat before a race," says trainer Arthur Lydiard, "you'd think they were worried about dying of malnutrition after 50 meters."

They never do, but Dr. Jean Mayer thinks they may feel that way if they aren't getting the 6,000 or more calories a day he recommends.

On the other hand, there are runners who find that they

can get by on as few as 1,200 calories a day. Famous runners' trainer Ernst Van Aaken also believes that less is more and that runners should keep a bottom line on calories, exceeding no more than 2,000 a day.

The bias toward running in this discussion of food calories is based on the fact that the best and the most research on the athletic diet has been done in this sport. And since most sports involve a certain degree of running, anyway, and none are more strenuous than running, the lessons learned have many applications elsewhere.

Of all the diet-related factors, reports the magazine *Runners World,* the one that seems to have the most dramatic effect on performance is reduced body weight. Specifically, fat beyond 10 percent of the ideal body weight, they say, is what slows you down. Therefore, fewer calories taken in means fewer miles are needed to burn that amount off.

A full-grown adult uses 1,500 to 1,800 calories daily to keep his basal metabolism purring. If you multiply 24 calories, one for each hour of the day, by the number of kilograms you weigh, you will arrive at the number of calories necessary to maintain your basal metabolism.

But then it becomes tricky. The range of energy needs is rangy to say the least, depending on the degree of activity in which the athletic body in question is engaged.

The variance in caloric expenditure from one sport to another can be mind boggling. For instance, some experts divide sport into two camps: endurance sports with higher energy cost, and sports of short duration and/or lower energy cost.

In Category A, there are such activities as long-distance swimming, soccer, wrestling, long-distance running, rowing, competitive skating, and skiing and gymnastics.

Category B includes archery, baseball, golf, tennis, short-distance skating and running, slow swimming, moderately vigorous cycling, and volleyball. You get the picture. If you don't, the charts in the Appendix should make it clearer.

Obviously, the caloric expenditures are larger for Category A than for Category B. But how much larger?

Ask yet another researcher and you will find that there are two sports camps, yes, but this time it's not the same two. Dr. Roy Rosenthal explains that caloric demands are variable because the same amount of energy invested in RE (risk exercise) and non-RE (nonrisk exercise) sports affects people differently. Non-RE sports exhaust, while RE sports exhilarate. Low-risk activities tend to get dull and tiring, while risk taking is exciting, in other words.[1]

Turning to Moretta and Turchetti, we learn,

> Normally, the individual in training requires 4,000 calories per day. For grammar or high school students, this should be adjusted to accommodate rapid growth rates. On the college level, it has been found that 5,000 to 6,000 calories are necessary for football and crew, a bit less for hockey, baseball, and track.

Over a two-hour period, a curler will expend approximately 1,000 calories. By comparison, two hours of tennis incurs a debt of 1,176 calories, and volleyball sets you back 700.

Any sort of exercise will set you even further back calorically if it's cold. The rule of thumb is that you can eat an additional 15 calories every day for each one-degree drop in temperature. A winter athlete sloshing around in the Arctic cold would need about 750 more calories a day than his counterpart in the Tropics, in other words.

Knowing the intensity of your sport will give you a better lead on figuring your nutritional caloric needs.

Walking, bowling, and golf are considered "light intensity" sports because they produce a pulse rate of 120 or less; jogging, tennis, racquetball, cycling, and hiking are generally considered sports of "moderate intensity," producing a pulse rate of 120 to 150; and "heavy intensity" sports include fast running, rapid swimming, and so on (pulse rate over 150).

Running is a real energy eater; 600–700 calories are needed to run 6 miles as opposed to 180 to run 1½ miles.

Or take swimming, ranked as the third most beneficial sport. East German swimmers, who are probably among the most intensively trained in the world, are given five meals a day for an average of 4,000 calories per each 70 kg. of body weight.

If you swam sixty strokes a minute for periods of forty hours, like Diana Nyad, you would need 12,000 calories a day or thereabouts, depending on your body type, to keep in caloric balance.

Marathon swimming burns up as many as 15,000 calories and 5 to 20 pounds, whereas swimming the crawl for us non-Nyad-type swimmers uses approximately 14 calories a minute.

An hour of fencing sets you back 600 calories, and gymnastics is good for 200–500.

Then there's cycling, considered second only to running in terms of health benefits.

Calories per minute expended on level ground are 5, 7, and 11, respectively, for speeds of 5.5, 9.4, and 13 miles per hour.

And while the average man may only require 3,000 calories a day, a cyclist averaging 30 to 60 miles per day may require twice that much to stay in weight balance.

In any discussion of energy, oxygen is the hero. It is the stuff that gives you an extra edge on the turf, track, or court.

Ernst Van Aaken, who ought to know, believes that oxygen outranks food as the most important ingredient in playing and winning. He says your oxygen pool is increased by distance walking and mountain climbing, riding a bike, skiing, and particularly endurance running.

Oxygen is needed in order to change the hydrogen in our bodies into water and energy.

Oxygen is the food for the work of the heart, brain, and other organs. So sensitive to a deficiency of oxygen is the brain that a few seconds without it are sufficient to bring on a blackout. Needless to say, insufficient oxygen can affect the levels of your game, and certain foods and types of nutrition strongly influence oxygenation of the organism.

What you are aiming for, say experts on energy-through-oxygen, is a pulse that doesn't rise above 130 under athletic stress. This is considered the most efficient breathing rate.

Although all of us contain enough stored energy to run, for instance, great distances, the speed of that running is limited by how rapidly we convey oxygen to the working muscles.

The respiration and the oxygenation of all the vital organs, and therefore your energy levels, depends to a great extent on the presence of vitamin F, the essential fatty acids. Another vitamin that keeps the oxidation-reduction system of tissue respiration in good repair is ascorbic acid, in ample doses.

You can improve your oxygen uptake considerably (and normalize your levels of iodine and potassium and stabilize your blood sugars at the same time) with some B_{15} in your daily diet. Or you could do some long-distance training at high altitudes.

The Tarahumara Indians are super athletes who burn up more than 10,000 calories on their daily runs, yet do it on a semistarvation diet by our standards. Speculates one observer, "Part of their energy comes from their highly adapted systems, developed by running every day of their lives in the thin air of the mountains."

And then there is *"ATP."* The high-energy compound must transform some of its energy into the useful work of drawing the muscle filaments together. This ATP must be replenished if you wish to have your muscles continue doing what they're doing. Because the supply of ATP in the muscle is small, this is accomplished by the healthy blood stream, which supplies the muscle with oxygen and nutrients, including glucose. The biochemical factories in the muscle cell then oxidize the glucose, utilizing the resulting energy for the reconstruction of ATP.

So more ATP would be helpful—that means a slightly higher fat intake. And so would a healthy blood stream, which is accomplished by applying as many of the principles set forth in this book as possible.

You are your own incredible energy machine. Tune it up and turn it on.

The Energy Connection, Part 2

Calories and the Overweight Athlete
"All people and nations eat too much and for this reason are poor performers."

—PAAVO NURMI, 1925.

Getting straight nutritionally usually involves getting skinnier. It is unfortunately true that most overweight problems are the result of being just a few calories per day out of balance. That is how Charles T. Kuntzleman, author of *Activetics* sees it. What he further sees is that it takes thirty-six hours of walking, seven hours of splitting wood or eleven hours of volleyball to lose one 3,500-calorie-pound of body fat. Taking three 15-minute walks a day, however, could result in a loss of a pound every fifteen days or twenty-four pounds in a year. "Never sit," says Kuntzleman, "when you can stand. The caloric difference is 10 calories. And get into the habit of pacing."

If you are on a rowing team, this is not very practical advice, but for other stand-up overweight athletes, it can be a helpful hint. As is the knowledge that if you are looking to exercise to drop a few pounds, swimming is a better choice than volleyball. The latter burns 3½ calories a minute, while doing the crawl eats up a full 14. And the energy expended during a half hour of squash, handball, or racquetball every day is the equivalent of 19 pounds of fat, which you would be carrying around at the end of a year if you hadn't been hitting the ball around.

And despite the common reputation of exercise as an appetite stimulant, it is actually the reverse that is true. According to Dr. Jean Mayer, nutrition and weight specialist, moderate physical activity decreases the appetite.

One of the most exciting studies of the connection between exercise and weight loss is cited by columnist Dorothy Harris.[1] It suggests that six hours after exercise you are still burning more calories than you would be if you had not exercised at all.

If you're fat-fat, maybe you should become a nut-nut. Cyclist-runner-writer George Beinhorn says, "When I tried a pure vegan (no eggs or milk) diet, using mainly nuts for protein, I immediately lost eight pounds more, though my caloric intake was about the same, and I was exercising less."

Or there is fasting, which, according to Gary Null of the Nutrition Institute of America, can result in a loss of one to three pounds each day, starting sometime during the first 10 days or so of a fast.

On the other hand, you may be the wrong weight because of food allergies. In that case, Dr. Newbold has an ideal diet, which is largely one of omission and which should help you lose weight or even gain weight if that, lucky you, is the problem. Some of the foods it excludes are: sugar, most sweets, barley, corn, milk and milk products, honey, and pastries, all foods that incite eating binges in food-sensitive individuals. Processed foods, in general, are verboten.

Supplements are generously included in Dr. Newbold's diet. "When I cut out certain vitamins from my own diet," says the author, "it is much harder for me to control my appetite. When I have my vitamin and minerals in near balance, food is not necessary to give me a feeling of force and strength. . . ."

Massive doses of ascorbic acid seem to afford coping power. Vitamin C can even help you lose if your new poundage is the result of food binges brought on by your food allergies.

Whether or not food allergies are at the bottom of being an overweight athlete *does* make a fat lot of difference. Studies show, for instance, that overweight athletes tend to develop tennis elbow more readily than their leaner partners. Fitness and fatness are not fellow travelers on the tennis court, track, or anywhere else.

Who, then, is actually helped by a little extra padding? Contrary to propaganda from some sports corners, the traditional obesity of weight lifters and the beef cakiness of football players seems to have no basis in augmented performance, says *Sportsmedicine* magazine. Ordinarily, the magazine continues, a sufficient amount of body fat seems always to be available. Overfattening may impair performance by increasing the inertia of the body and the energy cost of the performance.

Jogger and writer Hal Higdon adds, "Fat beyond 10 percent of body weight is what slows you down. If you don't believe that 5 pounds can make a difference, consider how fast you could run tomorrow if you had to carry a 5 pound weight on your back."

If reducing is your game, how and what should you lose?

One of the best weight-reduction tools seems to be the

open road. In a report on a sampling made by *Runners World* magazine of its readers, two out of every three reported losing weight doing what they liked to do best. The typical loss was between 10 and 20 pounds. Fifteen percent of the respondees reported losses of over 30 pounds.

If high mileage has low appeal for you, you might consider giving up meat. A Harvard-affiliated M.D., Dr. Hardinge, who completed a celebrated study of vegetarianism with Dr. Frederick Stare, concluded that nondairy vegetarians are 8 to 12 pounds lighter than milk-and-egg-eating vegetarians.

And Dr. Creig Hoyt notes, "It is a curious and yet unexplained fact that vegetarians can eat the same amount of calories as meat eaters and still gain much less weight." Despite approximately the same caloric intake and physical activities, vegetarians averaged 20 pounds less than the other two groups of meat, milk, and egg-eating men and women.

Or you could cut back on either fats and oils or protein.

A proponent of the first idea is Nathan Pritikin, a writer and runner. He says eating a 600-calorie-a-day diet, with calories largely derived from natural carbohydrates and as free of oils and fats as possible, leads to the loss of one pound every other day.

Proponents of the second notion say that losing weight comes easier if you increase your workouts and decrease the protein in your diet.

According to Dr. Gerald Combs, high-low swings in appetite can be correlated to high-low swings in amino acid levels in the blood stream. Eating your protein in a number of small, balanced meals throughout the day is an ideal appetite and weight regulator.

The dieting athlete, however, has problems that are somewhat different from those of the dieting nonathlete. It's important, for instance, to know what you can part with and what you can't afford to give away. One of the latter is water.

Its loss, alas, gives an appearance of rapid weight loss since a pound of sweat disappears ten times faster than a pound of fat. But it takes only one beer or two glasses of water to put it back. "Man generally relies on his thirst to control his body-fluid balance," says exercise physiologist David Costill. "Unfortunately, this mechanism is very poor, it appears, since after a large sweat loss, it may take days to redress an imbalance."

So the best way to guard against chronic dehydration and associated fatigue, mineral imbalance, and a false sense of weight loss is to check your weight each day before breakfast. If you're down 2 or 3 pounds from the previous day, you aren't short on fat. You're short on water, and that's not the loss you're after.

You could take a whack at your fat with what many experts consider an especially appropriate therapy for weight loss: juice fasting. Fasting on the raw juices of celery, watercress, and nettles, to name a few good raw ingredients, is especially effective. You should see dramatic results in three to four weeks.

You might arrive at your goal by upping your oxygen intake. There is considerable evidence that obese persons contain large amounts of hydrogen that they are unable to burn up because in an untrained body there is too little oxygen, and what there is can't be efficiently delivered. Burning up 1 gram of body fat—turning it into water and energy—requires 2,000 liters of oxygen, the equivalent of walking well over 100 kilometers.

Another way, reported in *Sportsmedicine,* in an article entitled "Weight Reduction Tools," is to create a deficit in your fat depot by a combination of diet and exercise. "The study indicates," says the magazine, "that if a person exercises during weight loss the loss of fat is greater and there is an increase in lean tissue." Persons losing weight by diet alone lose body tissue," which physiologist Creig Hoyt thinks is bad. "For the athlete trying to lose weight in order to improve his aerobic fitness, the best weight reduction plan is a gradual one of moderate calorie restriction. If you lose weight at a rate of greater than one-third pound per day, your muscular strength will decline due to this too-rapid loss."

This brings up another problem peculiar to the athlete: the whole problem of trained-on versus eaten-on fat. Increasing your "trained-on" fat in order to turn in peak performances is the result of long-distance training over many years (or the equivalent in persistent, consistent workouts in other sports), says Dr. Joan Ullyot, herself an M.D. and a distinguished marathoner. Such trained-on fat is an edge that is either earned by the acclimatized athlete or an edge with which you are born if you are a woman, since females tend to come naturally packaged with a slight surplus of fat, which explains their tendency to excel at pursuits requiring endurance, like distance running and swimming. Exercise has a definite and profound effect on fat, its amount, its distribution in your body, its utilization by your body's systems, and the extent to which it is used when you go into your act.

While the amount of fat stored in the muscle tissue is definitely related to an athlete's training, excess depot fat or "eaten-on" fat is something else again.

According to recent Swiss studies on the subject, well-trained runners had an average of 22.3 percent trained-on fat, while in lean runners not trained in distances the average was 10 percent.

Manipulations of diet, type, and amount of exercise can increase the effectiveness of the fat-burning system. And it also appears that consistent, persistent doing of what you do day after day improves your fat-burning system's overall effectiveness, especially when coupled with the proper diet, resulting in a better use of all nutrients, including fat.

The likelihood that you will win, place, or show at whatever you do decreases with each unsightly pound you add. "Obese persons," says the author of *Nutrition and the Athlete*,[2] "develop cardiovascular diseases about 80% more frequently than persons of normal weight and diabetes about 70% more frequently." On the other hand, the likelihood that you will stay obese after you've gotten into sports is less because, having gotten yourself into better than average shape, your engine idles at a lower rate. When you *do* exercise, you burn up lots of calories, but when you are not exercising, you use up fewer, and the appetite gets retrained right along with everything else.

According to diet authority Irwin Maxwell Stillman, no one should gain another pound after the age of twenty-five.

Diet, but do it right. "A wrong diet," warns Dr. Hans Kugler, "can make you age at ten to fifteen times the normal rate. That means if you diet wrong for one week you can do as much damage to your system as thirty weeks of normal aging would do. We interfere with hundreds of chemical reactions. We do serious damage to our systems; and that's exactly what happens when you go on one of those diets that limit you to one type of food only."

The two most important factors contributing to the rugged, robust health of the world's longest-living and highly athletic people studied by Dr. Alexander Leaf were a restricted diet and a high lifelong level of physical activity. Of the three tribes studied, the Hunzas, Abkahazias, and Viacamambas, *Sportsmedicine* magazine observed, "Their lives seem to be one long bout of exercise on lean rations."

So be it with you.

9 / *Special Cases*

Women and children last. They usually are in sports, sometimes for good reasons, sometimes not.

One recent instance of women coming in last occurred in Canada in a recent survey conducted by Dr. Donald Bailey, a physical education instructor at the University of Saskatchewan. But this time the kids finished first. The study, described as the most extensive assessment of fitness ever made in Canada, demonstrated that the least fit of all the groups were young women in their twenties. And teen boys scored the highest.

"The average American female begins a lifelong physical decline between the ages of 10 and 12," says Dr. Bailey.[1]

Obviously for every one of the women who is riding a bike these days, there must be two who are home reclining and declining. And more's the pity. A young woman who is inactive, warns Dr. Evelyn Gendel after studying a group of females between 17 and 25 at the University of Kansas, "pays a price in backaches, chronic fatigue, and menstrual difficulties." The myth that a woman is incapacitated by her monthly period is just that. Conditioning actually strengthens the back against the stress of menstrual flow.

Ditto the myth that exercise makes for unsightly muscles. Heavy muscles in actuality are a result of the male hormone androgen. Athletic women, in fact, lose fat more than they gain masculine muscle.

One sport in which they are doing just that is the physically draining sport of rowing, which is now flourishing among college women. "It's terribly exciting for women to see that they can be strong," says Connie Cervilla, captain of the Radcliffe crew, "to build their bodies as well as their minds. That's what being a woman is all about."

Being a woman is also about having certain things going for you and against you. For instance: The female knee is constructed wider than that of the male; the female has wider hips. She is also 20–25 percent lighter than the male, with a lower center of gravity and a shorter and narrower foot on a shorter leg. Women also have smaller lungs and slightly less breathing capacity. Considered minuses are that she also has a less dense bone mass than a male, shorter bones, and a faster calcium metabolism.

In a 160-pound man, the heart weighs about 1 pound and is about the size of his fist, but both male and female hearts are equally responsive to the effects of training. The average untrained woman's heart volume is 620 cc., while that of her untrained male counterpart is 730. Occasionally, a woman athlete is tested with a heart volume twice that of her untrained sister. So take heart.

A woman's mineral metabolism differs from a man in

ways that can make a difference in performance levels. Women, for instance, need 18 mg. of iron daily, while men require only 10. According to writer-runner Janet Newman, who looked into mineral matters, iron-deficiency anemia, just as they say in the ads, can be the reason why females are not the better half in sports. A woman between the ages of twenty and thirty has 5 percent less hemoglobin than her male counterpart. Since it is by fractions that everything is measured in sports, such a figure can be significant. Essentially, it means women's blood has a far smaller ability to carry oxygen, and the ability to carry oxygen is what it's all about.

Almost winning is the same as losing in sports. A chronic deficiency of anemia can bring your hemoglobin down to 50 percent efficiency. There may be a reason you feel played out before the play has begun. For reporter Newman, regular iron supplementation brought her hemoglobin up 10 percent in one week. But all iron isn't the same. You gotta shop around, as described in the discussion of supplementary minerals. The wrong kind could be worse than none at all.[2]

Why can't a woman in sports be more like a man?

Allan J. Ryan, III, editor of *Sportsmedicine* magazine, feels there is almost no sport in which a woman can't excel if she chooses: "With proper training women are fully capable of vigorous and demanding physical exercise, and they are not more susceptible pound for pound to injury, to serious or disabling injury, than men."

A woman has more stored fuel and less dead weight than her better half, a plus in sports in which endurance is the key to winning.

Trainer Ernst Van Aaken speculates that women not only have more fat, they have the enzyme systems to use it to good advantage. Which also means they hang on to their glycogen stores longer and are less frequently the victims of "hitting the wall," that state in competing (especially marathoning) when the fuel runs out.

Why do women excel where endurance is the factor? Because, says Dr. Van Aaken, of the way that they metabolize fat.

In running, for instance, the oxidation of fats is very important. The capacity to use that fat can be developed further by daily runs over long distances and the daily ingestion of 50 grams of foods rich in fats.

And how is the woman who exercises different from the one who doesn't?

For one thing, her body has a better fat-to-lean ratio. Dr. Jack Wilmore and his colleagues from the University of California at Davis report the relative fat percentage of adult sedentary women as being 28.1 percent, while an active group of female runners of comparable age and weight were only half as fat, with 15.2 percent. This is closer to the average college male's percentage of body fat.

Smaller leg bones, little feet, and narrower shoulders aside, women win because they try harder. According to America's top swim coach, Sherm Chavoor, "I'm convinced that girls can take more pain and suffering than boys. I know, for example, that Debbie Meyer trained harder than Mark Spitz."

The average woman is 23 percent muscle compared to 40 percent in her male counterpart, but sometimes it doesn't seem to matter a bit. Women swam so fast in the 1970 Olympics that by comparison Don Schollander's gold-medal time in the 1964 Olympics men's 400 meters would have only won him a bronze in the 1976 women's 400 meters.

"A woman has to do anything twice as well as a man to achieve credibility," agrees long-distance runner Kathy Switzer. This being the case, you need all the help you can get, so don't handicap yourself with a dumb diet.

And there's nobody for whom a dumb diet could be dumber than for your kids.

According to Ernst Van Aaken, "Children between five and fourteen whom I examined had much higher endurance quotients on the average than untrained adults." A greater heart capacity, he believes, explains this for the most part.

A seven-year-old in good health has a faster recovery ability than a world-class athlete, he adds. A child reaches his normal pulse values in just a few minutes because his organism immediately switches over to "play-pulse levels after exertion. . . . The endurance capacity of the child and adolescent is constantly being underestimated by both sports doctors and coaches." [3]

Indeed, young preteen girls are often superior to boys of the same age group in running because of their lean frames and low weight.

But Van Aaken warns against "sports emphasizing . . . explosive muscle functions . . . which cause oxygen debt, something the young body incurs with reluctance and which if repeated too often can survive only at the cost of organic damage. . . ."

He heartily advises running. "It is just children who are born long-distance runners. Any healthy boy or girl is able to run as much as three miles at a moderate pace. The play of children is nothing more than a long-distance run. Because in a couple of hours of play they cover many kilometers with several hundred pauses. The play of children is a primal form of interval training."

And what is it that provides proper food fuel for the smaller sports?

Extra protein is kidstuff. While no increased protein beyond the RDA is needed by someone exercising vigorously, in this case, the muscles are actually growing bigger as well as stronger. These mini-athletes need a healthy input of first-grade proteins. Since the brain is growing and the immunity system is flowering, disastrous results can come from cutting back the protein in a young athlete's diet.

So, too, are extra calories true kid stuff.

While a college student involved in football or crew would require about 5,000–6,000 calories and nearly that much for hockey, baseball or track, the figure should be adjusted a bit downward for high-school and grade-school athletes.

The caloric needs for the grade-school athlete go something like this:

ages 9–12, 33 calories per pound per day; ages 12–15, 31 calories per pound per day; ages 15–18, 25 calories per pound per day.

And why does the young athlete tend to satisfy those caloric needs at Burger King or the nearest Coke cooler?

The culprit, suggests James White, physical education professor at the University of San Diego, is probably the snack shack, a phenomenon familiar to parents everywhere. The high stress that is the inevitable lot of the Little Leaguer, coupled with a ready availability of junk food, puts the growing athlete in "double jeopardy," as White sees it. "Unbuffered by protein, the gulps of sugar and caffeine which are the prime ingredients of cola-type soft drinks are especially hard on an immature metabolism. Worse, they are often hard to refuse because they are offered free by exploitative soft drink companies."

Which often leads to or compounds a weight problem.

If one parent is fat, the child has a 40 percent chance of being fat. The Youth Fitness Council, under President Kennedy, found that among two thousand kids tested, ages four to twelve, less than 10 percent had reached a satisfactory level of physical fitness, and 25 percent were overweight.

So what can you do in addition to following the general advice on vitamins, foods, on what to admit and omit in the youngster's diet.

What else can you do for a tired teen-ager, an under-weight sandlotter?

For starters, try bee pollen, which reputedly stimulates a quick rise in hemoglobin in children and also builds weight and strength.

Wheat-germ oil works its wonders on kids, too. According to trainer Chris Miles, the feeding of fifteen 6-minim capsules of the oil each day to active ten to thirteen-year-old athletes resulted in significantly reduced reaction times.

In another study in which three groups of boys age seven through fourteen were fed milk, wheat germ, or wheat-germ oil and then given a "hop test," the oil-fed group outhopped the others by a full twenty-eight hops.

Another way to give your kid an edge is to lace his diet with honey. In a study run by a Swiss M.D., Dr. P. Wessen, daily doses of honey were fed to one group of children, but not to two control groups, which only got placebos instead. The group using honey each day surpassed the others on several counts: higher blood count, more normal weights, more energy and improved appearance.[4]

Another special case is the older athlete. If you still want to be going like forty when you're sixty, hear this.

"A decrease in the efficiency of your organs in old age," says Dr. Hans Kugler, is "directly related to a decreased and faulty protein synthesis in your body." Dr. Kugler says two of the consequences of a diet deficient in essential amino acids (protein) are: "the maintenance of all organs and body processes will be hampered (and) several hormones will not be formed since they depend upon proteins for satisfactory synthesis. . . ."

Man is at his best shape in the decade before twenty-five, says New York internist Dr. Donald Tomkins. His muscles are firmest, and his body is most efficient at utilizing nutrients. Peak health begins to decline when the body process called anabolism (cell growth) is overtaken by the opposite process, catabolism (cell death). Cells start dying faster than they are replaced, and muscle is replaced by fat.

Some observers say that a sharp deterioration occurs in neuromuscular function during the 50s and 60s. Exercise can considerably retard this process, which is something you have already observed in yourself if you are past your prime and still "at it."

Specifically, what is longevity-promoting exercise? According to Dr. John Bullock, a physiologist and exercise-aging authority at the New Jersey Medical School in Newark, isotonic exercises that tax the heart most are the best age-delayers. This would mean swimming, tennis and skiing are better bets than walking.

If you doubt that adopting a few dietary practices that extend life might improve the quality of your sporting life, consider Dr. Kugler's statement, "If you could prevent only 10 percent of the aging factors in your system and undo another 10 percent of the damage already done, your maximum life expectancy would be approximately 280 to 340 years."

Dr. Kugler points out that just by feeding laboratory mice a combination of vitamin E, sulphur amino acids, and other antioxidants, it was possible to extend their lives 66 percent.[5]

One way to prevent middle-aged spread, if not middle age itself, is to run 5,000 or 6,000 miles a year as the American Medical Joggers do and try out the diet that helps some of them do just that:

Take about a gram of vitamin C for each 6 miles and take visible amounts of yeast and wheat germ oil for their content of B complex and the unsaturated fats (EFAs) . . . .

Avoiding highly refined foods is recommended: sucrose, starch, saturated fats, and distilled alcohol. Otherwise, a balanced diet with fresh fruit, raw vegetables, moderate red meat (fish instead of meat for many meals), plus the wheat-germ oil (or other vegetable oils that are not hydrogenated), yeast (or yogurt), and vitamin C (or an orange for each mile).

Dr. Thomas Bassler, the organization's president, further adds that marathoners over forty should take 1 gram of ascorbic acid for every 6 miles they run to prevent injury to ligaments, tendons, and bones. That's a formula that can be adapted to your benefit even if you aren't Boston Marathon bound.

In the opinion of Paavo Aorola, the ultimate secret of staying young is the secret of staying healthy, accomplished by what he calls his "Optimum Diet," the cornerstone of which is the consumption of up to 80 percent of your food in its raw and natural state. Raw nuts and seeds and sprouted grains, he contends, are the Fountain of Youth foods.

To Doctors Frank and Passwater, however, the key is a combination of vitamins in big hefty doses with nucleic acids. In lieu of a youth drug, such a combination has more than once been shown to improve dramatically the youthfulness and longevity of lab rats.

"After a person passes his prime, the amount of enzymes eliminated in his urine and feces begin to decline. It continues decreasing until he dies. Older persons should take special care to preserve what is left of their enzyme potential and add to it through raw foods and enzyme concentrates."

Note that the enzymes in the lining of the intestinal tract

needed for the digestion of sucrose lose their effectiveness with age, too, which may be why sweets are now causing you a rum tummy.

Any older athlete might want to consider the power-through-protein plan that put Bobby Riggs in the winner's circle in a matter of seven weeks of intensive food training.

Nutritionist Rheo Blair tells of the foods of fitness that did it: "Many meat dishes (only from organically grown cattle), fertile eggs, certified raw milk, raw milk cheese, protein-bolstered sugarless milk shakes. . . ."

So to improve your performance chemistry if you're pushing fifty or sixty begin by examining the calorie, enzyme, and protein content of your diet.

And remember, extra pounds through extra calories can hold you back considerably. A very large energy and food need in adolescence may dwindle to a very modest need indeed by middle age. Between twenty-five and thirty-five, basal needs alone decrease by 50 calories a day, and by fifty-five they have declined by 150 calories a day. If you fail to make the necessary reduction, you could be hauling around 10 more pounds than you'd like to on the courts, course, track, or field. If you want to really take off, take it off.

10 / How to Be Your Own Jock Doc

Combining Foods

All the foods for fitness in the world won't do you a whit of good if you don't combine them properly.

Food combining is an important part of eating for fitness. You are in reality not so much what you eat as what you digest. Lots of often-partnered foods don't combine.

For instance, wheat germ and honey, the authors of *Food for Fitness* point out, is a lousy food combination from your stomach's point of view. Similar pre- and postgame combinations probably don't get digested and therefore produce only a small part of the energy they should.

What is a correctly combined meal, anyway? The greatest authority on this is probably Herbert Shelton, who has been at it since 1928 and still runs his aptly named Health School in San Antonio, Texas, between writing books about how to practice what he preaches. Dr. Shelton is quick to point out that animals, for instance, eat very simply and do almost no combining at all. Squirrels, in other words, do not have to have everything from soup to nuts to consider themselves well fed. Nuts alone seem to fill the bill.

The reasons are as simple as the uneaten parsley on your plate: There is no value to be derived from foods that are not digested. Proper combining also provides a protection against poisoning since improperly digested foods only waste or spoil in the digestive tract. Shelton's experience is that what we called "allergy" is in many cases "protein poisoning," caused by improperly digested proteins that turn to putrefactive waste and cause angry reactions.

Hygienists say that a cardinal rule is to take only one starch at a meal and add no sugars to it. Otherwise, fermentation is almost inevitable.

Eating foods that contain apparently opposing elements—cereal, for instance, contains both starch and protein—is not the same thing as eating foods of opposing characters. Bread and cheese are an example. "Nature," says J. H. Tilden, author of a classic book on the subject of food combining "never produced a sandwich."

Different foods require different mediums in which to be digested, which is why it is not a sound idea physiologically to combine, for instance, starch and protein. This only results in a traffic jam since the starch must be digested first and the protein must wait. If you care enough, you will eat your protein first and your starch last, assuring that the protein will digest in the lower end of the stomach while the starch digests at the upper end.

Your stomach can only do a limited amount of gear shifting to digest what you give it.

Water should not be drunk with your meals. It tends to dilute stomach juices and wash away those enzymes needed to digest the food. Starches should be eaten dry and salivated well before swallowing.

Have a smallish salad at noon with your starch for the day and a larger salad at night with your protein input for the day; that's one suggestion from food-combining authorities. If you have your water fifteen minutes before you lunge into either repast, you may not have to reach for the antacid at all. Speaking of which, remember that acidity is a state that tends to encourage ill health, and that state is the one that meat eating puts your body in. Other do's and don'ts: Flesh foods require the most amount of gastric juice, while milk requires the least. And don't eat them together. Eat only one concentrated protein at a meal. Eggs and milk are out, as are meat and milk.

If you want your stomach to be empty before the big game, remember that it is a particularly poor idea to combine protein and fat. Fatty meats slow digestion down to a walk and inhibit protein digestion for two hours, maybe longer. Fat digestion is considerably bettered when it is combined with green vegetables. A vegetable salad with a cup of cashew nuts, for example, is A-O.K. with the food physiologists. So is steamed asparagus and a plate of peanuts, another case of coupling fat and greens. Or cottage cheese on top of beet greens. Get the idea?

Another combination likely to set back digestion and stomach-emptying times is sugar plus any kind of protein. If you're still a coffee hound and use cream and sugar in it, beware. That "twofer" delays the overall digestion of the meal for several hours. Sugars, because they are not digested in the mouth or stomach, tend to ferment when eaten with protein because they must wait until the protein is digested separately. All sweet foods tend to slow digestion down, which sheds some light on the "don't spoil your appetite with sweets before dinner" mandate.

Contrary to the common assumption that acids help in

the digestion of protein, the two are better eaten separately. Acid actually interferes with the digestion of protein. Exceptions are nuts and rich cheeses, which do not decompose as quickly as other proteins because of the generous amounts of fats that they contain. Their digestion is not seriously delayed by acids.

Acid-starch combinations also are indigestible.

Fruits should be eaten solo. They are only digested in the small intestine, and they are not digested at all if they meet with other food groups on the way down. Fruit meals are best taken at breakfast time, and sweet fruits should not be paired with acid ones.

Finally, melons and milk should always be eaten apart from all other foods. Milk combines poorly with other foods, although it combines better with acid foods than with any other group, if nothing's going to stop you from having your cheese with oranges on top.

In the matter of desserts, you guessed it. The advice is to skip them entirely. Most pies, cakes, and ice creams, either because of their high sugar content or combination of starch-protein-acid ingredients, are out.

To simplify all this, here is raw-food vegetarian Karen Whyte's food-combining formula:

Eat one meal of fruit, another of vegetables, and a protein meal along with a leafy salad.

And if it still seems too complicated, there's always fasting.

Beyond food combining and digestion lies assimilation.

If you don't assimilate your food properly, you run into one of the major causes of fatigue. We are all biochemically different, and the old saw about one man's meat is quite literally true in the case of metabolism and assimilation.

Your oxidation rate is a significant factor in not just whether you win or lose but whether you have enough energy to play the game at all.

The speed rate at which the body turns food into energy

is called the oxidation rate. Everybody's oxidation rate has a rhythm all its own (similar to the "biochemical individuality" that nutritionist-author Roger Williams writes about).

A slow oxidizer will be unable to burn sugar fast enough to utilize a heavy fat-protein intake. This person burns carbohydrates inefficiently, and a diet too high in fat or protein causes trouble. Neither fat nor protein can be turned into energy if sugar is not being broken down normally.

So there are low- and high-performance foods suited best to slow oxidizers and fast oxidizers.

The fast oxidizer is one who burns sugar unusually fast, with a consequent increase in the way he uses up acetate, the richest of all the energy-producing intermediates. This type of person suffers during cold weather unless he increases his fat and lowers his carbohydrate intake.

Fast oxidizers react rapidly and poorly to coffee, and starch and sugar combinations, whereas slow oxidizers get a lift from such a meal, which increases the rate of sugar utilization in the brain by virtue of its caffeine content.

Nor are one oxidizer's supplements another's. The person who burns food too slowly needs a different set of foods than a person who burns foods too rapidly, and they even have different vitamin-mineral needs.

The moral? Know your type if you would increase your energy. Your doctor can determine where you stand by the appropriate lab tests.

To understand your stomach, it is essential to know something about enzymes. These may be defined as physiological catalysts.

There are various stages in the digestion of foodstuffs, and each stage requires the action of a different enzyme. The enzymes can do their jobs only if the enzymes before them have done theirs. It is all a matter of the right key in the right lock.

Enzymes are special proteins that promote vital chemical changes; food fuses without which you would starve to death no matter how much you ate because your body would be unable to turn food into energy and living cells. There are over six hundred different types of enzymes, and none of them duplicates the work of the others, amazingly enough. Perhaps the most important one is the one you've probably heard about: hydrochloric acid. An insufficiency of this enzyme may result in the body's inability to liberate iron and translate it into a form the body can use.

The word "enzyme" means to ferment or to leaven (from the Greek) and is practically synonymous with foods for fitness. The fittest foods contain the most enzymes: fruits, honey, milk, nuts, and berries, all in their uncooked state. Plus fermented vegetables, fermented breads, milks, and so on.

Exogenous enzymes, from outside the body, are contained in the following foods: brewer's yeast, raw honey, papaya (contains papain, which helps digest protein), kelp, rose hips, and double-threat foods like sauerkraut, soured milks, soured pickles, etc.

In general, enzymes should be used to repair and remodel worn and neglected body parts. Food enzymes from raw food predigest the food; it spares the body a load of work. Unfortunately, they rarely get a chance to fill this function because, thanks to the enzymeless cooked meals we eat, they are kept busy just digesting all this processed input. As a result, theorize the experts, illness enters the picture. And amino acids are consumed in great quantity to enable the body to adequately make enzymes, says Rheo Blair, Bobby Riggs's remake man and nutritionist.

In addition to outside sources, our bodies have a limited enzyme-manufacturing ability. If enzymes are not provided from raw, fresh food, the body is forced to use up more of its own enzymes faster, so that by age forty you may not have as much fuel for your sporting life as you ought. That's especially true if you've been eating bad foods for any length of time. Then to the rescue should come supplements such as pancreatic enzymes, hydrochloric acid, and comfrey-pepsin.

"It is not unreasonable to use enzyme extracts on a regular basis in the same way that people take vitamins. . . . Vitamins can't do any work, hormones can't do any work, without enzymes," says Dr. William Kelly.

Indeed, when you get to the point where you can't make certain enzymes, as another expert points out, "then your life ends." That's how important *enzymes* are!

How can you supplement your diet, then, with enzymes, especially if you're over forty and are convinced that they are important? You can promote this salutory predigestion process by taking chewable tablets or powders along with your meals. Of course, if you are eating an all-raw meal, this supplementation isn't necessary. Pick the plant concentrate rather than the pancreatin-type of supplement because they work longer. And avoid the coated tablets that are designed to bypass the stomach and work in the small intestines.

What does digestion have to do with athletic achievement or underachievement? More than you might imagine.

Good digestion means more normal tissue changes throughout the body. It results in a general improvement in all the functions of life; the whole process of blood making, for example, is interconnected with digestion. Which brings up another aspect of the mechanics of eating, the timing of meals. Timing is as important as what you eat in the opinion of many experts. The scheduling of your food breaks might have an especially beneficial effect on your energy levels. "Never eat a big breakfast. Never, until at least two to three hours after you get up" is an idea whose time has not exactly come among more conventional nutritionists, but sports nutritionists embrace it as they embrace the liquid meal because it works. It spares the stomach for a while.

"You should get up and drink a lot of fruit juices or water and get out and exercise until your body is cleansed. And you have earned your breakfast," says Paavo Airola.

A few more rules:

1. If you want the total reserves of your body to be available for athletic activity, don't eat for three to four hours before you plan to go into action. This will allow the digestive system to clear itself.
2. Forty-eight hours before events or games, eliminate high-fiber and bulky food items and any very sweet foods, that is, all raw fruit (except bananas and oranges), all raw vegetables, seedy vegetables, whole-grain products, nuts and popcorn, gravy, jams, preserves.
3. Remember that a tennis match, a road race, a diving competition, even a friendly game of paddle tennis can be a mild to moderate stress situation for you. If so, you will require two to four hours longer than usual to digest your food. A liquid meal may be the solution for you.
4. Since stress induced by athletic activity doesn't disappear that rapidly, postgame eating should be postponed for an hour. Drinking fruit juices for several hours is a safer bet than tossing off a hamburger or a victory dinner even if you think you owe it to yourself. When your dithers have definitely subsided, you can consider a light meal, that is, about 500 calories' worth.
5. Overeating won't improve your game, so don't overload your circuits. This practice has now even been pushed to the front rank of reasons why you might get cancer, according to *New York Times* reporter Jane E. Brody.
6. People in the know, like biochemist Richard Passwater, recommend five or six small meals in preference to the conventional big three.

Not only does input and output matter but the speed at which foods enter and leave your system affects your performance, too.

Here, in general, is a run-down on transit, or stomach-emptying, times.

Meat: remains about two and a half hours in the stomach. Pork takes longer, ham requires eight hours, and sweetbreads and pork sausage longer yet.

Eggs: come and go faster than meat, but scrambled eggs linger longer.

Vegetables: Peas and carrots and green beans are quickest to go.

According to Professor Macareg of the Philippines, x-ray studies of athletes fed a liquid meal before competing showed that the stomach was empty in two hours and digestion completed in four hours, with little nausea, indigestion, etc.

You, too, might switch to a pourable meal both before and after you play. Just make sure it is raw, real, and digestible.

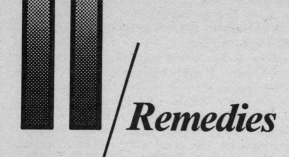

11 / *Remedies*

Last year more than nineteen million sports-related injuries were brought into medical offices, the result of nonprofessional sports activities.

If you were among the millions injured, maybe you could have done some of the doctoring yourself. Now that sports medicine is with us, preventive sports medicine can hardly be far behind.

Since $4.5 billion is already being spent remedying the ills that arise from medically dispensed drugs, the sooner you learn how to take your own tennis elbow in hand the better.

Here is a roundup of remedies and preventive remedies for sports people:

- To prevent body odor, make sure your diet runneth

over with leafy greens. Ample doses of chlorophyll-rich foods seem to prevent perspiration odors.

- Likewise, the distress of low-blood-sugar attacks can be offset by a healthy intake of green juices: parsley, lettuce, chard, beet greens, etc. Dilute with water and drink at half-hour intervals.
- If you are allergic, avoid overtraining, says jock doc George Sheehan. It makes allergies worse and can cause glandular enlargement. If you're a runner and a frequent victim of right-side pain, Dr. Gabe Mirkin (also a runner) suggests that switching the emphasis in your diet from breads and other starches over to fruits and vegetables helps. This works as a cure for constipation, too.
- Feeling dopey? Mix some Gotu Kola leaves in with your salad, or take a cup of Gotu Kola tea for extra alertness.

Many aerobic sports perform what author Roy Ald calls the "Guardian Functions." Running and many other aerobic sports are preventives for a host of complaints. When you run, promises Ald, you are defending yourself against the common ailments related to the digestive system: ulcers, colitis, diabetes, constipation. Also, he says, you are protecting yourself against ills of the circulatory system, including hypertension, cardiac and arterial disorders, and disfunctions of the motor system, because you are strengthening your motor nerves, frame, joints, and ligaments. You're probably blocking the onset of joint-disabling ills such as neuritis, neuralgia and backache, too.

If you are stumbling around in a state of mesotrophy (half health), maybe you need a sweat fix. Or a fever fix.

Besides the cleansing process that the sauna, hot tub, fever, Turkish bath, steam bath, etc., prompts, "overheating also accelerates healing and restorative capacities," according to Paavo Airola, a Finn from the land of

700,000 steam baths. It stimulates all the metabolic processes, and stems the growth of virus or bacteria, he says.

What if you don't have a Finnish sauna in which to finish off the good works that your exercise has started? A "combination of heavy exercise or exhausting, perspiring games, with swimming in a pool or the ocean can substitute for a Finnish sauna," Airola says.

As for nature's "wonder drugs," pollen is literally the bees' knees. If pollen can cure radiation sickness, imagine what it might do for your heel spur or your trick knee. Pollen literally makes a perfect poultice for swellings, according to Charles W. (Doc) Turner, head trainer at Long Island University and is nature's medicine for injured knees and elbows. He has personally treated 189 of them with his pollen poultice and in the last two years reports success with all but two. Doc's formula goes like this:

> Pollen pellets are dissolved in warm tap water to form an infusion. A towel is dipped in the mixture and applied to the injured area. Turner said he had seen swelling go down a half-inch in 20 minutes as a result of the treatment. In the comments he has collected from patients, most also report a great decrease in pain and discomfort.[1]

There certainly seems to be a need for knee medicine. According to a poll of one thousand dedicated runners, two-thirds of them had suffered injuries serious enough to lay them up for two weeks, the most common being "runners' knee." Other frequent problems were stress fractures, inflamed Achilles tendons, and bone spurs. According to L. A. Baker, D.V.M., of California, who has also treated many injured athletes, the mineral manganese is helpful in preventing Achilles-tendon injuries. Its deficiency, he writes, was first noticed as a cause of slipped-tendon disease in turkeys.

A natural remedy for runners' heel spurs, the result of calcium deposits, is to eliminate the cause, which some chiropractors say is the result of drinking homogenized pasteurized milk. The next step, to take certain prescribed amounts of bonemeal tablets (for calcium) and liquid phosphoric acid to dissolve the deposits, is a solution that has worked for some sufferers.

If you're over thirty-five, your problem may be higher up, however. It is estimated that 50 percent of the country's players over that age will have tendonitis at one time or another. It is rare, says Dr. Nirschl, assistant professor of orthopedic surgery, Georgetown University School of Medicine in Washington, to see anyone under thirty with tennis elbow. But does anything really help the condition?

Dr. Plagenhoef, professor of biomechanics at the University of Massachusetts, offers this opinion: "I have to say one thing about your cortisone. I have never yet met one person that cortisone has helped. It relieves temporary inflammation. If you resume play too early, the pain comes right back. If you resume waiting, you have rested it long enough, anyway."

Leg cramps are a problem common to both runners and tennis players. Indeed, to any athlete whose sport involves more than a minimum amount of two-legged hustle. What is the cause? In most cases, says Dr. George Sheehan, a runner himself, the cause is salt depletion. You may be losing more fluid than you are replacing during exercise. How to tell? Weigh yourself before and after the event to discover your total fluid loss. Then you should replace this loss with some suitable solution.

If fluid replacement is not the problem, you might experiment with carbohydrate loading (see Special Diets) which gives twice the normal sugar content to the muscles and often prevents cramping. Each gram of glucose also corresponds to 2.7 grams of water. Since more glucose is stored by the liver with this diet, there is less chance of low blood sugar levels, too.

It may be useful to know what a cramp is in the first place. Finley P. Gibbs, writing in *The Best of Bicycling,* says, "A muscle cramp is simply a muscle that has contracted but failed to relax when the nerve stimulation has ceased." He adds that "it is interesting to note that energy from ATP is also required for relaxation to occur."

Says Dr. L. Lotzhof, writing in the *Medical Journal of Australia,* "I have tried Vitamin E with remarkable success on approximately 50 patients suffering from muscular cramp." A daily dosage of 300 mg. was found sufficient to control most cramping.

And if breaking rather than cramping is your problem, Adelle Davis reports, "Coaches who insist that the athletes have orange juice daily and cod liver oil in some form have reported fewer broken bones and other serious injuries during the season."

Sprains of the ankle, foot, and toe, if they aren't exactly brought on by salt abuse, can be cured by its near omission in your diet, according to the *American Family Physician* magazine. Reduced salt intake gets rid of excess body fluids, and such accumulation at the site of an injury is what causes all that pain.

On the other hand, if you practice real preventive medicine you may not have to worry about troubleshooting; you won't have any troubles. Witness Dutch marathon runner Aad Steylen, who, after two years on a natural diet, went the whole route, became a vegetarian, and nourished himself with whole cereals, brown rice, raw vegetable salads, fruit, nuts, and vitamin E-rich oils. He told the editors of *The Runners Diet,* "I have had hardly any infectious diseases, tendon, cartilage, joint or muscle injuries. I trace this back to my natural diet which provides the body with the necessary nutritional and building substances. These are just as important as training."

End of commercial.

But if you do get sick despite a diet of wheat germ and yogurt, put pollen on your list of internal medicines.

"From their bellies comes a liquor that is medicine for man," goes a saying in the Koran. And that liquor is pollen. It is reportedly helpful for a wide range of maladies including asthma, hayfever, anemia, and diarrhea.

According to Dr. Rene Chauvin, pollen seems to possess an antiputrefactive factor, too. His patients suffering from diarrhea and similar problems improved on pollen, and so did their digestion and assimilation.

Honey is a honey of a medication, too, as well as valuable for treating athletically inflicted wounds, cuts, bruises, and burns. For a test run, spread some honey on your next cut before bandaging and see how speedily you mend.

Or try B_1, the energy vitamin, by mouth and see how fast you recover. Recent studies indicate it has great therapeutic potential, which makes sense since B_1 plays a vital part in the synthesis of the body's protein. The vitamin also helps relieve side effects from antibiotics.

Or take C and see.

According to the *Rodale Book of Vitamins,* football players at Louisiana State University found that while vitamin supplementation (especially vitamin C) had no effect on the number of bruises and injuries they received in the game, those who had supplementation recovered 23 percent faster.

To promote healing of all kinds, Linus Pauling, in *Runners World Magazine,* advises a larger intake of vitamin C plus some vitamin E in doses of at least 400 I.U. Dr. Paavo Airola also recommends ascorbic acid, which turns out to be probably the cheapest, safest, wide-spectrum, all-purpose, over-the-counter remedy of them all.

Taken in advance of spurts of exercise, ascorbic acid also prevents muscular stiffness.

Another remedial aid for faster healing of injuries is B_{15}, especially when coupled with extra doses of protein, which is the way the Russian coaches do it.

Garlic is a curative with an almost disconcertingly rapid effect. Thirty drops of garlic-oil concentrate have been known to completely knock out all symptoms accompanying the flu. And Paavo Airola reports that studies in the United States, Russia, France, and Germany have employed garlic in treating everything from flatulence to high blood pressure. To remove the odor and improve its potency, you can "cure" your cure by doing what the Russians do: store crushed fresh garlic for twenty months or more in a large vat, then extract the juice. Take small, daily doses.

Just how do you administer garlic, whether or not you home cure it? You might take it as part of a "liver flush," which is sort of a salad dressing without the salad: Simply crush two healthy buds of garlic, fork-blend with freshly squeezed lemon juice and olive oil, and down the hatch.

Herbs in general are side effect free, inexpensive ways of dealing with athletic ills. They did, after all, make up as much as 80 percent of our drugs as recently as the 1800s.

Which echoes Dr. Hans Kugler's recipe for maintaining a healthy blood-sugar level "simply by eating foods high in protein."

And pangamate (B_{15}), too, says Dr. A. V. Lesnichy, writing in *Problems of Endocrinology* in 1968, helped prevent a lowering of blood-sugar levels.

"Regarding sports-related injuries and recovery, it is important to take the nucleic acid-rich diet but also minerals, particularly manganese, which helps in recovery from ligament injuries. Vitamin C is also helpful. . . ." So says anti-aging expert Dr. Benjamin Frank.

Another solution to ills emanating from the games people play is fasting. The reason fasting may bring quick relief to a number of problems is that it not only frees the digestive organs of some of their labors, but it removes allergic irritants which you have been unaware were the root of your ongoing discomforts.

Certainly it is one of the better and safer solutions to that broad category of ills that *Runners World Magazine* calls "internal disturbances."

Digestive malfunctioning is certainly not bettered by the taking of antacid tablets and alkalizers of any description. This is especially true for the athlete, because they create an environment in the stomach that is hostile to the absorption of calcium, a critical nutrient in the sports diet.

You might, of course, prevent "internal disturbances" completely if the cause is (1) eating the wrong foods at the wrong time; (2) eating too much too soon before playing; (3) eating too much in general.

It is wise to remember that the body is capable of living off its own resources for long periods, and the significant wisdom of precontest fueling up is dubious at best. Every ounce of food increases the body's load, as any seasoned athlete will warn you.

Appendix I

RECIPES

You've heard of a bicycle built for two?

Well, here's a bicyclist's Carrot Flan for Four, courtesy John and Gay Wilcockson and reprinted by permission of *Bike World Magazine.*

CARROT FLAN FOR FOUR

whole wheat pastry case
1½ lbs. carrots
1 tbsp. brown sugar or
  honey

2 oz. sweet butter
tomatoes
1 tbsp. corn oil
parsley

Wash and slice carrots. Boil in a minimum of water, then mash them by hand or electric blender. Add 1 tbsp. brown sugar or honey, 2 oz. sweet butter, and a pinch of salt.

Spoon the mixture into a pastry case, 8–9 in. in diameter. This case is made of whole-wheat dough and should be pricked and baked "blind" for 15 min. prior to making the flan. Once the mixture is in the case, you may want to arrange some sliced tomatoes on top.

Brush on 1 tbsp. corn oil and bake for 15–20 min. at 350°. Before serving, sprinkle with chopped parsley.

MOCK VEAL
(for four or more)

And another, which, if the Wilcocksons didn't invent as vegetarians, they would certainly approve of.

¾ lb. fresh carrots	1 cup cooked brown rice
1 cup raw peanuts (skinless)	2 eggs
1 medium onion	salt to taste

Grind carrots, nuts, and onion; mix all. Pack in oiled 9 × 5 loaf pan. Bake about 45 min. at 375°.

RELIEF PITCHERS

Mineral and enzyme-rich thirst quenchers for energy before, during, and after the match.

Nut Milk

1 cup water	6 pitted dates
1 cup orange juice	⅓ cup sunflower seeds (hulled)

Blend well.

Fruit Milk

3 large mashed bananas	1 whole, peeled and pitted lemon, juiced

Liquidize. Add a little water if necessary.

Fruit Milk Plus (Iron-Rich)

4 oz. pineapple juice
4 oz. prune juice

1 raw egg
1 tbsp. brewer's yeast

Blend together.

Double Nut Milk

½ cup almonds, ground
½ cup cashews, ground
1 tbsp. liquid lecithin
1 tsp. honey
pinch of salt

2 cups hot water
½ cup soy milk powder
2 cups cold water

Blend first six ingredients 1 min. or more; add soy milk powder and 2 cups cold water. Blend to mix well; add enough water to make ½ gal.

Avocado Milk

½ ripe avocado
1 tbsp. fresh lemon juice
1½ cups tomato or V-8 juice

dash liquid red pepper
1 cup alfalfa sprouts

Blend everything. A liquid meal for two.

JOCK JERKY

½ cup undergerminated
  cornmeal
1 cup unsweetened apple
  sauce

pinch cayenne
pinch sea salt

Mix all ingredients. Spread clear plastic wrap over one large baking sheet and secure the corners with tape. Preheat oven to approximately 150°.

Using a spatula, spread the fruit-meal mixture thinly over the plastic wrap. Set in oven with door ajar and let oven dry for 2–3 hrs. Turn oven off and let "jerky" continue to dry for an additional 24 hrs., or longer if necessary.

Carefully peel the "leather" from the wrap into a long roll. Wrap in a new swatch of clear wrap and use scissors to snip off bite-sized pieces as needed for quick energy.

SUPER CEREAL

½ cup raw wheat germ
½ cup raw oat flakes
2 tbsp. brewer's yeast
2 tbsp. sunflower seed
2 tbsp. flaxseed

2 tbsp. sesame seed
2 tbsp. bran
1 tbsp. chia seeds (optional)
1 tbsp. honey
a few raisins and sprouts

Grind above in blender, mixed with water from sprouts or milk and a banana, or pour on fruit juice or one of the special milks from the Relief Pitchers recipes.

HOMEMADE FRUCTOSE

1 cup dried figs/and or
dates (Other dried fruits
may be used, but these
taste the best.)

Dry the fruits further, preferably under a hot sun or in a low oven until they are extremely dried, even hard. Break into small pieces and put into blender of nut mill and grind till you have pulverized them finely. Store in a tightly closed container. Delicious on cereals, toast, fruit.

SPORT SALT #1

½ cup fresh herbs
1 cup sea salt

Choose any completely dry fresh herb or herbs that go
well together—dill and sweet basil, parsley and rosemary,
sage and thyme. Whirl in blender with sea salt for 2 to 3
min. Then spread on a stainless-steel cookie sheet and dry
in oven at 120° for 1½ hr. When cool, funnel into glass salt
shakers and label.

SUPER SPORT "SALT" #2
(A salt free high-mineral seasoning)

This is based on combining any of the following:

parsley flakes	*mustard seed*
onion flakes	*dried watercress*
garlic flakes	*caraway or poppy seed or*
bell pepper flakes	*sesame*
celery seed	*brewer's yeast flakes*
dill seed	*assorted dehydrated*
dried mushroom flakes	*vegetable flakes*
cumin seed	

Combine any of the above ingredients in any amounts
you desire. Pretoast the cumin seed and mustard seed and
sesame, and use only half as much of these as of any other
herb in the mixture. Pulverize everything in seed mill or
blender.

SOFT FROZEN *YOGURT*

(Note: recent taste tests run by a *New York Times* food
writer indicated that the best-tasting plain yogurt for
freezing was Continental.)

2 cups of fresh plain yogurt

¼ cup unpasteurized honey; add a little chopped honeycomb for extra luxury

¼ cup date sugar or fruit sugar (both available at your local health food store)

½ cup of freshly squeezed lemon juice

1 teaspoon grated lemon peel, optional

Combine ingredients in blender or food processor or beat by hand until smooth. Adjust the sweetening (it should be on the tart side), pour into a prechilled freezer can, and follow the manufacturer's instructions for making ice cream, allowing if necessary an extra 30-45 min. for best soft-whipped results.

JOCKS BLOCKS

5 figs

1 tsp. vitamin C or rose hip powder

3 eggs

¼ cup of cottage cheese

2 tsp. vanilla

1 tsp. lemon

1 cup grated carrots

2 oz. ground almonds

2 oz. ground sunflower seeds

2 tsp. cinnamon

1 tsp. nutmeg

2 tsp. honey (optional)

2 tsp. carob powder

2 tsp. chopped walnuts (optional)

Blend figs first; then add and blend eggs and cottage cheese. Fold in rest of ingredients. Bake in oblong baking dish approximately 1 hr. at 350°. Cool 15 min. and cut into 1-×-3-in. blocks. Refrigerate.

SUPER BOWLS

Soups to soup you up? Dr. Ralph Bircher has spent a lifetime comforting people, athletes among them, with apples, potatoes, and other high-quality proteins. "Potatoes," he says, "contain barely 2 percent protein but of the highest quality equal to that of eggs. In combination with small amounts of egg protein, potato protein is of the very highest value. . . . Test subjects eating potato as their sole source of protein remained healthy and strong for five and a half months. . . ."

Doubtless you would remain even healthier with some garlic added, so here they are together to work their special effects:

Garlic Potato Broth

1½ qt. potato peel broth	½ bay leaf
peels from 6 unsprayed potatoes	1 head garlic, broken into cloves and peeled (about 16 cloves)
herbs	
egg shells	¼ tsp. thyme
1½ tbsp. olive oil	pinch of sage

Put potato peels in a pot with water to cover twice and any herbs you favor, plus eggshells or bones to add calcium. Add a bit of lemon juice, bring to a boil, and simmer, covered, 30 min. Strain. Combine broth with other ingredients and simmer slowly for 30 to 45 min. Discard the garlic cloves and the bay leaf. Serve with sprinkling of finely minced hard-boiled egg on top, or beat in 1 raw egg as for egg drop soup.

The possibilities are now endless. For a fine, clear soup, serve the hot broth as is with some cooked noodles or rice. Fresh vegetables, such as thinly sliced carrots, sweet peas, cubed potatoes or sliced zucchini may be added and simmered until tender for another soup. Try it also with little dumplings. This broth is excellent, of course, for sauces, risotto, cream soups, and many other recipes that call for consomme.

Potassium Broth

This popular alkaline broth is based on the Hippocrates formula, which he recommended to all those who felt "under par."

1 cup finely shredded celery, leaves and all	1 qt. water
1 cup finely shredded carrots	1 cup thick tomato puree
½ cup shredded spinach	1 tsp. vegetable salt
1 tbsp. chopped parsley or chives	1 tsp. honey
	parsley or chives

Put all shredded vegetables into a quart of water. Cover, bring to a boil, reduce and cook slowly for 30 min. Then add tomato puree or tomatoes, vegetable salt, and honey. Let cook for 5 min. more. Strain and serve. A sprinkle of chopped parsley or chives will add vitamins, minerals, and color. You may also include any one of your favorite vegetables or herbs.

VITA-TURF

No, don't stay off the grass, grow it. This kind isn't fattening, illegal, or immoral, and it should raise both your health level and the level of your game.

Sprouted seeds are wonder foods with a wonder food inside them. Chlorophyll, the inner ingredient, has been described as "concentrated sun power." It is credited by those who should know with increasing and sustaining the normal functions of the heart muscle and raising the basic nitrogen-exchange levels.

kernels of whole wheat　　　*some clean dirt or good*
whole rye　　　　　　　　　*potting soil*
whole radish
cress or alfalfa seeds (or a
　mixture)

Take a large planter with good drainage and fill ⅔ full of good dirt. Scratch rows with the blunt end of a pencil, leaving ½ in. between rows, and sprinkle seeds in fairly close proximity. Cover with dirt, water generously, and cover planter with plastic wrap until seeds begin to sprout. Remove cover and put your planter in sunlight until the "grass" comes up. If planted in rich soil, this special "lawn" will be rich in natural vitamins, minerals, enzymes, and trace elements like chlorophyll. Clip the grass with scissors and sprinkle the clippings in your salad, soup, juice, or dessert. Then get another plot of Vita-Turf going. You can keep various kinds of "appetite-appeasing" mini-lawns growing all year.

Appendix II
CHARTS

WHAT GOOD DOES YOUR GAME DO YOU?

	JOGGING	BICYCLING	SWIMMING	SKATING (Ice or Roller)	HANDBALL/ SQUASH	SKIING (Nordic)	BASKETBALL	SKIING (Alpine)	TENNIS	CALISTHENICS	WALKING	GOLF*	SOFTBALL	BOWLING
Physical Fitness Cardio-respiratory endurance (stamina)	21	19	21	18	19	19	19	16	16	10	13	8	6	5
Muscular endurance	20	18	20	17	18	19	17	18	16	13	14	8	8	5
Muscular strength	17	16	14	15	15	15	15	15	14	16	11	9	7	5
Flexibility	9	9	15	13	16	14	13	14	14	19	7	8	9	7
Balance	17	18	12	20	17	16	16	21	16	15	8	8	7	6

	JOGGING	BICYCLING	SWIMMING	SKATING (Ice or Roller)	HANDBALL/ SQUASH	SKIING (Nordic)	BASKETBALL	SKIING (Alpine)	TENNIS	CALISTHENICS	WALKING	GOLF *	SOFTBALL	BOWLING
General Well-being Weight control	21	20	15	17	19	17	19	15	16	12	13	6	7	5
Muscle definition	14	15	14	14	11	12	13	14	13	18	11	6	5	5
Digestion	13	12	13	11	13	12	10	9	12	11	11	7	8	7
Sleep	16	15	16	15	12	15	12	12	11	12	14	6	7	6
Total	148	142	140	140	140	139	134	134	128	126	102	66	64	51

Source: Reprinted with permission of *Medical Times* (May '76), © 1976 by Romaine Pierson Publishers, Inc., 80 Shore Rd., Port Washington, N.Y. 11050.

VITAMIN UPPERS
What Pangamate (B₁₅) and Tocopherol (E) Can Do for You

Comparison of Vitamins B_{15} and E

MECHANISMS

Vitamin B_{15}	Vitamin E
Oxidative metabolism	Antioxidant
Lipotropic	Antiradical
Methylation	Enzymatic (not well established)

FUNCTIONS

Vitamin B_{15}	Vitamin E
Extends cell lifespan	Extends cell lifespan

* Ratings for golf are based on the fact that many Americans ride a golf cart. If you walk your golf, the physical-fitness value moves up appreciably.

Improves blood oxygenation
Stimulates immune response
Involved in energy transport
Detoxifies pollutants
Involved in protein synthesis
Liver protecting
Normalizes fat transport
Provides methyl groups
Speeds recovery from fatigue
Regulates blood levels of steroids

Improves blood oxygenation
Stimulates immune response
Involved in energy transport
Detoxifies free radicals
Involved in heme synthesis
Platelet protecting
Membrane stabilizer
Anticlotting
Prevents excessive scarring

DISEASES (Common to both vitamin B_{15} and vitamin E)

Heart diseases
Intermittent claudication
Aging
Senility
Diabetes
Gangrene
Hypertension
Hypercholesterolemia
Glaucoma

Cataracts
Cancer protection
Air pollution protection
Muscular dystrophy
Liver necrosis
Arthritis
Asthma
Emphysema

(Diseases specifically treated with only one of the two vitamins)

Vitamin B_{15}
Alcoholism
Drug addiction
Autism
Minimal damage brain dysfunction
Schizophrenia
Cirrhosis
Hepatitis
Jaundice
Allergies
Dermatitis
Iritis
Mild poisoning
Neuralgia
Sciatica
Cachexia

Vitamin E
Encephalomalacia
Hemolytic anemia
Steatitis
Embryonic degeneration
Exudative diathesis
Pancreatic atrophy
Menopause
Prostatitis
Burns
Fertility

Xanthomatosis
Strabismus
Neuritis

Natural Sources of Pangamate (Vitamin B_{15}) (milligrams per 100 grams of food)			
Rice Bran	200	Wheat Bran	31
Corn Grits	150	Barley Grits	12
Oat Grits	106	Wheat Flour	10
Wheat Germ	70		

Source: Reprinted with permission of *Let's Live* magazine, August 1977. Compiled by Richard A. Passwater, after Teleydy-Kovats et al., 1970.

HOW ATHLETES' PERFORMANCES HAVE IMPROVED OVER THE PAST 80 YEARS

MEN'S OLYMPIC EVENTS

Track and Field:	1896	1928	1972	1976
100-meter dash	12.0	10.8	10.14	10.06
200-meter dash		21.8	20.00	20.23
400-meter dash	54.2	47.8	44.66	44.26
800-meter run	2:11.0	1:51.8	1:45.9	1:43.5
1,500-meter run	4:33.2	3:53.2	3:36.3	3:34.2
5,000-meter run		14:38	13:26.4	13:24.7
10,000-meter run		30:18.8	27:38.4	27:40.38
High jump	5-11	6-4½	7-3¾	7-4½
Shot put	26-9½	52-¾	69-6	69-¾
Long jump	20-10	25-4¼	27-¼	27-4¾
Swimming:				
100-meter freestyle	1:22.2	0:58.6	0:51.22	0:49.99
400-meter freestyle		5:01.6	4:00.27	3:51.93
1,500-meter freestyle		19:51.8	15:52.58	15:02.4
4 x 200-meter freestyle relay		9:36.2	7:35.78	7:23.22

WOMEN'S OLYMPIC EVENTS

Track and Field:	1896	1928	1972	1976
100-meter dash		12.2	11.07	11.08
800-meter run		2:16.8	1:58.6	1:54.94
High jump		5-2½	6-3½	6-4
Discus throw			191-2	218-7
4 x 100-meter relay		48.4	42.81	42.55
Swimming:				
100-meter freestyle		1:11.0	0:58.59	0:55.65
400-meter freestyle		5:42.8	4:19.04	4:09.89
200-meter breaststroke		3:12.6	2:41.71	2:33.35
4 x 100 medley relay			4:20.75	4:07.95
100-meter backstroke		1:22.0	1:05.78	1:01.83

Source: From the *Miami Herald*

"In general, the rise in athletic performance can be attributed in many cases to increased exercise together with improved food habits . . . ," Autti Ahlstrom, assistant professor of Public Health, the University of Tampere, Finland.

SUGARFULL

Food	Portion	Approximate Sugar Content in Teaspoonful of Granulated Sugar
Berry pie	1 slice	10
Cherry pie	1 slice	10
Sherbet	½ cup	9
White icing	1 oz.	5
Ginger ale	6 oz.	5
Soda pop	1 (8-oz. bottle)	5
Chocolate cake	1 (4-oz. piece)	10
Macaroons	1	6
Chocolate eclair	1	7
Donut (glazed)	1	6

Fudge	1-oz. square	4½
Hard candy	4 oz.	20

IPC figures compiled by makers of Calcident tablets.

The approximate amounts of refined sugar (added sugar, in addition to the sugar naturally present) is hidden in popular foods.

SUGARFREE

Food	Food Energy per Pound (calories)
Almonds	2685
Bread (whole wheat)	1125
Dates	1415
Figs (dried)	1290
Honey	1333
Peanut butter	2616
Raisins	1410
Maple syrup	1485
Soy	1576
Dried apples	1190
Carob	1440
Peanuts	2255
Rice	1610
Walnuts	2640

Food—Natural Sugar—Starch Content

	Percentage		Percentage
Blackberries	12.5	Carrots (raw)	9.3
Raspberries	13.8	Onions (raw)	10.3
Oranges	11.2	Lima beans	19.3
Apricots	12.9	Peas (cooked)	12.1
Bananas	23.	Boiled sweet potatoes	27.9
Dried dates	75.4	Baked white potatoes	22.5
Dried figs	68.	Kidney beans	16.4
Grapes	15.5	Sweet corn	20.2
Peaches	12.	Peanuts (roasted)	23.6
Plums	12.9	Pecans	13.
Prunes	71.	Almonds	19.6
Dried raisins	71.2	Cashews	27.1

SPORTS WITH LARGE ENERGY COSTS *

Basketball	Long-distance skiing
Gymnastics (especially apparatus)	Long-distance swimming
Handball	Middle-distance running
Hockey (ice and field)	Mountaineering
Long-distance rowing	Paddleball
Long-distance running	Soccer
Long-distance skating	

SPORTS WITH MODEST ENERGY COSTS *

Baseball	Short-distance running
Bowling	Short-distance skiing
Canoeing, slow or moderate speed	Short-distance swimming
Cycling, slow or moderate speed	Skating
Diving	Ski jumping
Golf	Tennis
Rowing, slow or moderate speed	Volleyball

A BREAKFAST FOR CHAMPIONS
(Wrong Way)

One cup of instant breakfast drink (imitation-orange flavored)

Ingredient	Delivers
Sugar	Adds calories; offers temporary burst of energy
Citric acid	From chemicalized fermentation process; adds a high acid flavor; may damage teeth and bone enamel

---

* Roughly 4,000–5,000 calories a day, depending on hours of training spent, body weight, and size.

* Roughly 2,000–3,000 calories if practiced no more than one hour daily.

Ingredient	Delivers
Flavor	Chemically prepared flavor from real or artificial sources to duplicate the natural flavor of the orange
Gum arabic (vegetable gum)	A plant gum that acts like a mucilage; may prompt intestinal irregularities or allergic response
Monosodium phosphate (also known as sodium biphosphate)	An emulsifier and sequestrant that binds and inactivates minerals in the body; high sodium content
Potassium citrate (also known as sodium citrate)	Buffer or acidifier, a sodium salt of citric acid; acts as the sequestrant above; high sodium content
Calcium phosphate	Refined and purified chemical to prevent caking; caustic; may cause allergic intestinal distress
Vitamin C	Usually synthetic (may be a coal-tar derivative)
Cellulose gum	A natural plant gum, usually from a vegetable source; may cause allergic or intestinal reaction
Hydrogenated coconut oil	A saturated fat that may predispose to cholesterol atherosclerosis build-up in arteries; adds "body" to the beverage

Ingredient	Delivers
Ferrous sulfate	Iron oxide reduced to a powder by the chemical addition of hydrogen; if strong enough, may be poisonous to children; may also cause liver damage
Artificial color	Adds the "look" of orange juice
Vitamin A	Usually synthetic (may be a coal-tar derivative)
BHA preservative (butylated hydroxyanisole)	A coal-tar product, used as an antioxidant; may have cancer-causing properties

BREAKFAST FOR CHAMPIONS
(Right Way)

One cup of pure orange juice

Nutrient	Amount	Delivers
Water	88%	Maintains proper body temperatures used by all hormones and body systems
Calories	110	Provides true energy for vigor and strength
Protein	2 grams	Builds, maintains, and repairs all body tissues; supplies energy; helps form antibodies to fight infection; contributes to the body's fluid structure

Nutrient	Amount	Delivers
Carbohydrates	26 grams	For real energy; helps the body use fats efficiently for body warmth; aids digestion by adding bulk
Calcium	27 mg.	Helps functioning of muscles, nerves, and heart; builds bones and teeth
Iron	.5 units	Pairs with protein to make the hemoglobin that carries oxygen to all body cells; aids cells in using oxygen and creating energy
Vitamin A	500 units	For healthy skin and eyesight; prevents night blindness; helps keep mucous membranes of mouth, nose, throat, and digestive tract healthy
Vitamin B_1 (Thiamine)	.22 mg.	Needed for proper function of heart and nervous system and energy production
Vitamin B_2 (Riboflavin)	.07 mg.	For healthy skin; prevents sensitivity of eyes to light; needed to build and maintain healthy body tissues
Niacin	1 mg.	Works with enzymes to convert food to energy; aids nervous system; prevents appetite loss

Nutrient	Amount	Delivers
Vitamin C	124 mg.	Keeps bone, teeth, blood vessels healthy; helps tooth formation; builds resistance to respiratory ailments; prevents fatigue
Potassium	460 mg.	For cell fluid balance, normal nerve-impulse conduction, and muscle contraction; regulates acid-alkaline balance
Magnesium	22 mg.	Relaxes nerves, promotes cell growth, and activates enzymes; helps form new proteins
Phosphorus	43 mg.	For healthy bones and teeth; needed by every cell and for the metabolism of carbohydrates

SALT-FREE *

Food	Amount	Sodium
Apple	⅓ lb.	1
Asparagus	4 spears	1
Bran (raw)	¼ cup	1
Corn	1 ear	trace
Cornmeal	1 cup	2
Cucumber	6 slices	2
Eggs	1	1
Orange juice	1 cup	3
Peanuts	1 cup	8
Tomatoes	1	6
Wheat flour	1 cup	4

* Or nearly so. Trace amounts of naturally occurring sodium appear in many, perhaps most foods. But that sort of salt is not the culprit.

SALT-FULL

Bacon	2 slices	153
Beans, lima, canned	1 cup	401
Beef, corned	3 oz.	1,491
Chicken pot pie	1 pie	932
Corn flakes	1 cup	251
Frankfurter	1	499
Pizza	1 slice	525
Potato chips	3 oz.	840
Soup (chicken, vegetable, onion, from dry mix)	1 cup	1,030
Ketchup	1 tbsp.	156
Baking powder phosphate	1 tbsp.	1,230
SAS	1 tbsp.	1,198
tartrate	1 tbsp.	874
Mustard, brown	1 tbsp.	352

(In non-salt-using societies, daily sodium intake may be as low as 800 mg. The average American diet averages between 4 and 10 grams.)

"The huge amounts of salt in the average American diet might well be the key to the escalating incidence of hypertension, edema, and the shortening of life that results from all these conditions...."

NATIONAL ACADEMY OF SCIENCES

HERBAL RENEWAL FOR THE ATHLETE
(Herbs as nutrients)

Vitamin A	Alfalfa, dandelion, okra
Vitamin B_1	Bladderwrack, fenugreek, okra
Vitamin B_2	Fenugreek, saffron
Vitamin B_{12}	Alfalfa, bladderwrack

Vitamin C	Burdock seed, calendula, capsicum, elderberries, oregano, paprika, parsley, rose hips, watercress
Vitamin D	Watercress
Vitamin E	Alfalfa, bladderwrack, dandelion leaves, linseed, sesame, watercress
Vitamin K	Alfalfa, chestnut leaves, shepherd's purse
Niacin	Alfalfa leaves, blueberry leaves, burdock seed, fenugreek, parsley, watercress
Rutin (part of the bioflavonoid complex)	Buckwheat, rue, paprika
Calcium	Arrowroot, camomile, chives, coltsfoot, dandelion root, nettle, sorrel, okra pods
Iodine	Bladderwrack
Iron	Burdock root, meadowsweet, mullein, nettle, parsley, strawberry leaves, watercress
Magnesium	Carrot tops, dandelion, kale, meadowsweet, mullein, okra, parsley, peppermint, watercress, wintergreen
Phosphorus	Garlic, chickweed, sesame, sorrel, licorice root
Potassium	Birch bark, carrot tops, camomile, clomfrey, dandelion, fennel, mullein, nettle, parsley, peppermint, primrose flowers, savory, watercress, yarrow
Sodium	Chives, fennel seed, meadowsweet, nettle, okra pods, sorrel, watercress

Chapter Notes

CHAPTER 1
1. *Let's Live* magazine, November 1975.
2. *Food for Fitness,* see Bibliography.

CHAPTER 2
1. Ruth Adams, *Did You Ever See a Fat Squirrel.* Emmaus, Pa.: Rodale Press, 1972.

CHAPTER 3
1. Roger J. Williams, *Nutrition in a Nutshell.* New York: Doubleday, 1962.
2. In a letter to the author.
3. John L. Kent, *Science Digest,* July 1977.
4. *Herald of Health,* February 1976.
5. Jacqueline Verrett and Jean Carper, *Eating May Be Hazardous to Your Health.* New York: Anchor Press, 1975.
6. Ernst Van Aaken, *Van Aaken Method.* Mountain View, Ca: World Publications, 1976.
7. *American Journal of Clinical Nutrition,* June 1976.
8. *Consumer Reports,* March 1978.
9. J. Daniel Palm, Ph.D., *Diet Away Your Stress, Tension & Anxiety; The Fructose Diet Book.* New York: Doubleday, 1974.
10. Beck and Hedley, *Honey and Your Health.* New York: Bantam Books, 1971.
11. Barbara Cartland, *The Magic of Honey.* Moonachie, NJ, 1970.

CHAPTER 4

1. W. D. Currier, *Let's Live* magazine, August 1977.
2. Henry Bieler, *Food is Your Best Medicine*. New York: Vintage Books, 1965.
3. *Let's Live* magazine, June 1977.
4. *Chemical and Engineering News* (Vol 52, No. 25, p. 5, 1974).
5. *National Enquirer*, January 3, 1978.
6. *Herald of Health* magazine, February 1976.
7. *Let's Live* magazine, March 1977.
8. Richard Passwater, *Supernutrition*. New York: Dial Press, 1975.
9. *Let's Live* magazine, May 1976.
10. Edward R. Pinckney and Cathey Pinckney, *The Cholesterol Controversy*. Los Angeles: Sherbourne Press, 1973.
11. Karen Cross Whyte, *The Original Diet*. San Francisco: Troubador Press, 1977.
12. ———, *The Complete Sprouting Book*. San Francisco: Troubador Press, 1973.
13. H. L. Newbold, *Meganutrients for Your Nerves*. New York: Peter H. Wyden, 1975.
14. *Encyclopedia of Healthful Living*. Emmaus, Pa.: Rodale Press, 1960.
15. *Herald of Health*, January 1977.
16. *Let's Live* magazine, February 1976 and August 1977.
17. *The New York Times*, Feb. 6, 1977.
18. *Swedish Medical Journal*, Vol 58, No. 36, 1961.
19. Nauka Press, Moscow, 1976.
20. *Health Survival Digest*, Vol 2, No. 2, 1977.

CHAPTER 5

1. In a letter to the author.
2. *Nutrition in a Nutshell.*
3. Ludwig Prokop in the European journal *Condition.*
4. *Health Survival Digest*, Vol 2, No. 2.
5. Rosenberg, Harold, *The Doctor's Book of Vitamin Therapy*. New York: Putnam, 1976.
6. Richard Passwater, *Supernutrition*. New York: Dial Press, 1975.

7. *Scandinavian Journal of Clinical and Laboratory Investigations,* Vol 17, No. 3, 1965.
8. *Bestways Magazine,* January 1976.
9. Ludwig Prokop, *Runners World,* July 1973.
10. Consumer Product Safety Commission. According to a report by Harald Taub in *Let's Live* magazine, April 1975.
11. Dorothy V. Harris, *WomenSports* magazine, Dec. 1977.
12. Rosenberg, *op. cit.*
13. Fred Klenner, Reidsville, North Carolina, physician of whom H.L. Newbold says "probably knows more about the clinical use of ascorbic acid than anyone else in the world."
14. Joseph J. Morella and Richard J. Turchetti, *Nutrition and the Athlete.* New York: Mason/Charter, 1976.
15. *Psychodietetics,* E. Cheraskin and Dr. W. M. Ringsdorf, Jr., with Arline Brecher. New York: Stein and Day, 1974.
16. Professor of Biochemistry at Loma Linda University School of Medicine. *Prevention,* October 1976.
17. *Family Circle* magazine, October 1975.
18. *Prevention,* February 1977.

CHAPTER 6

1. Richard Pardee, *Let's Live* magazine, May 1977.
2. *Harper's Bazaar,* April 1975.
3. *Harper's Bazaar,* April 1975.
4. *Family Circle* magazine, November 15, 1977.
5. Bergstrom and Hultman, *The Physician and Sportsmedicine,* magazine, January 1976, see Bibliography.
6. Pardee, *op. cit.*.
7. *Runner's World* magazine, August 1976.
8. *Let's Live* magazine, August 1977.
9. *Physician and Sportsmedicine* magazine, January 1976.
10. *Nutrition Today,* Vol 3, No. 2, June 1968.
11. *Vegetarian Times,* May-June 1977.
12. *Organic Gardening and Farming* magazine, May 1977.
13. Per-Olaf Astrand and Kaare Rodahl, *Textbook of Work Physiology.* New York: McGraw-Hill, 1970.
14. Henry G. Bieler, see Bibliography.
15. George Beinhorn, *Food for Fitness.* Mountain View, Ca.: World Publications, 1975.

16. *The Physician and Sportsmedicine* magazine, January 1976.
17. *The Physician and Sportsmedicine* magazine, March 1977.
18. Van Aaken, *op. cit.*
19. *Let's Live* magazine, June 1977.
20. Herbert M. Shelton, *Food Combining Made Easy.* Dr. Shelton's Health School, San Antonio, Tex., 1975.

CHAPTER 7

1. Charlotte Holmes, *Herald of Health,* September 1975.
2. *National Enquirer,* June 28, 1977.
3. *Nutrition Reports International,* May 1974.
4. Van Aaken, *op. cit.*

CHAPTER 8 (Part I)

1. *Family Circle,* October 1975.

Part II

1. Dorothy V. Harris, *WomenSports* magazine, October 1977.
2. Morella and Turchetti, *op. cit.*

CHAPTER 9

1. *Family Circle* magazine, October 1975.
2. *WomenSports* magazine.
3. Van Aaken, *op. cit.*
4. P.E. Norris, *Everything You Want To Know About Honey,* New York: Pyramid Books, 1970.
5. Hans J. Kugler, *Slowing Down the Aging Process.* New York: Pyramid Books, 1973.

CHAPTER 11

1. *New York Times,* February 6, 1977.

Selected Bibliography

Airola, Paavo O., *Health Secrets from Europe*. New York: Arco Publishing Co., 1972.

Anderson, Bob and Henderson, Joe, *The Runners Diet*. Mountain View, Ca.: World Publications, 1972.

Astrand, Per-Olaf and Rodahl, Kaare, *Textbook of Work Physiology*. New York: McGraw-Hill, 1970.

Atkins, Robert C. and Linde, Shirley, *Dr. Atkins' Super Energy Diet*. New York: Crown Books, 1977.

Beinhorn, George, *Food for Fitness*. Mountain View, Ca.: World Publications, 1975.

Bieler, Henry G., *Food Is Your Best Medicine*. New York: Vintage Books, 1965.

Davis, Adelle, *Let's Eat Right*. New York: New American Library, 1970.

Gerber, Ellen W.; Felshin, Jan; Berlin, Pearl; Wyrick, Waneen, *American Woman in Sport*. New York: Addison-Wesley, 1974.

Jacobson, Michael, *Nutrition Scoreboard*. New York: Avon Books, 1974.

Kugler, Hans J., *Slowing Down the Aging Process*. New York: Pyramid Books, 1973.

Leonard; Hofer; Pritikin, *Live Longer Now*. New York: Grosset and Dunlap, 1976.

Morella, Joseph J. and Turchetti, Richard J., *Nutrition and the Athlete*. New York: Mason/Charter, 1976.

Newbold, H. L., *Mega-Nutrients for Your Nerves*. New York: Peter H. Wyden, 1975.

Passwater, Richard, *Supernutrition*. New York: Dial Press, 1975.

Rodale, J. I., *The Complete Book of Vitamins*. Emmaus, Pa.: Rodale Press, 1966.

Rosenberg, Harold, *The Doctor's Book of Vitamin Therapy*. New York: Berkley Publishing Co., 1976.

Royald, *Jogging Aerobics and Diet*. New York: Signet, 1968.

Shelton, Herbert M., *Food Combining Made Easy*. Dr. Shelton's Health School, San Antonio, Tex., 1951.

Smith, Nathan J., *Food for Sport—1976*. Palo Alto, Ca.: Bull Publishing Co., 1976.

Ullyot, Joan, *Women's Running*. Mountain View, Ca.: World Publications, 1976.

Van Aaken, Ernst, *Van Aaken Method*. Mountain View, Ca.: World Publications, 1976.

Verret and Carper, *Eating May Be Hazardous to Your Health*. New York: Anchor Press, 1975.

Wade, Carleton, *Fact-Book on Fats, Oils, Cholesterol*. New Canaan, Ct.: Keats, 1973.

Waerland, Ebba, *Rebuilding Health*. New York: Arco Books, 1972.

Whyte, Karen Cross, *The Original Diet*. San Francisco: Troubador, 1977.

Williams, Roger J., *Nutrition Against Disease*. New York: Bantam Books, 1973.

Index

Also available from
STEIN AND DAY/ *Publishers*

THE OFFICIAL EATING TO WIN COOKBOOK:
Super Foods for Super Athletic Performance
Frances Sheridan Goulart

DR. MARCHETTI'S WALKING BOOK
Albert Marchetti, M.D.

A DICTIONARY OF SYMPTOMS
Joan Gomez, M.D.

HAVE YOUR BABY, KEEP YOUR FIGURE
M. Edward Davis, M.D. and Edward Maisel

THE TRUTH ABOUT WEIGHT CONTROL:
How to Lose Excess Pounds Permanently
Neil Solomon, M.D., Ph.D., with Sally Sheppard

PRIME TIME:
Getting More Out of It After 35
Morton Hunt and Bernice Hunt

THE NO MORE BACK TROUBLE BOOK:
Relief and Prevention
Edited by Edith Rudinger
Adapted by William T. Talman, M.D.

THE SKIER'S YEAR-ROUND
EXERCISE GUIDE
Thea Dee Slusky, R.P.T.

THE WOMAN GOLFER'S CATALOGUE
Jolee Edmondson

BACKPACKING
A Complete Guide to Why, How and Where
Lee Schreiber and Editors of *Backpacking Journal*

CAMPING
A Complete Guide to Why, How and Where
Andrew Carra and Editors of *Camping Journal*

MOUNTAIN CLIMBING FOR BEGINNERS
Mike Banks

Ask your bookseller!